Emergency Medicine

THE INSIDE EDGE

Emergency Medicine

THE INSIDE EDGE

PHILLIP M. STEPHENS, DHSc, PA-C

Assistant Professor
Campbell University School of Medicine
Southeastern Regional Medical Center
Emergency Medicine Residency Program

Adjunct Faculty, Doctorate of Health Sciences Program
College of Graduate Health Studies
A.T. Still University

Associate Provider Site Director
Southeastern Regional Medical Center
Department of Emergency Medicine

JEFFREY A. KLEIN, MD, FACEP

Assistant Professor
Campbell University School of Medicine
Southeastern Regional Medical Center
Emergency Medicine Residency Program

GINA S. STEPHENS, DNP, FNP-BC

Associate Faculty University of Phoenix

Senior Associate Provider
Southeastern Regional Medical Center
Department of Emergency Medicine

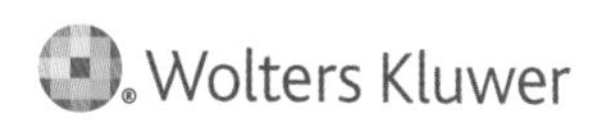

Philadelphia • Baltimore • New York • London
Buenos Aires • Hong Kong • Sydney • Tokyo

Acquisitions Editor: Sharon Zinner
Product Development Editor: Ashley Fischer
Editorial Assistant: Alexis Pozonsky
Marketing Manager: Rachel Mante-Leung
Production Coordinator: Sadie Buckallew
Design Coordinator: Teresa Mallon
Manufacturing Coordinator: Beth Welsh
Prepress Vendor: Newgen Knowledge Works Pvt. Ltd., Chennai, India

9 8 7 6 5 4 3 2 1

Printed in China

Library of Congress Cataloging-in-Publication Data
Names: Stephens, Phillip M, author. | Klein, Jeffrey A. (Jeffrey Allen), 1969- author. | Stephens, Gina S., author.
Title: Emergency medicine : the inside edge / Phillip M. Stephens, Jeffrey A. Klein, Gina S. Stephens.
Description: First edition. | Philadelphia, PA : Wolters Kluwer, [2019] | Includes bibliographical references and index.
Identifiers: LCCN 2018024856 | ISBN 9781496386021 (paperback)
Subjects: | MESH: Emergencies | Emergency Treatment | Handbooks
Classification: LCC RC86.7 | NLM WB 39 | DDC 616.02/5—dc23
LC record available at https://lccn.loc.gov/2018024856

LWW.com

RRS1807

Contents

Contents

Contents

Preface

Evidence-based medicine (EBM) is the integration of the best known scientific evidence with clinical experience. Bridging the gap between the latest research and clinical application is always a challenge. This text is designed to bridge this gap.

This is a powerful text in the hands of a trained medical professional. It is purposely concise. Rather than focusing on background information or pathophysiology, the text is designed for efficient application of the best evidence.

Clinicians can quickly review each heavily researched topic with its succinct format. Foundational key information is found under the "General" heading. Necessary workup information is found under the "Evaluation" heading. Treatment options are listed under the "Management" heading. Each option is not simply the author's opinion but is based on the latest best evidence. The references for each recommendation can be easily accessed as well.

You will find the most common issues encountered in emergency medicine. You will also find vital topics such as backboard clearance, drug diversion, and laceration care. Topics such as organophosphate poisoning, carbon monoxide toxicity, and ethylene glycol exposure are less commonly encountered but when you need the information, you need it quickly and concisely.

Charts that are required on a daily basis are at your fingertips. Having in your pocket pediatric vital signs, ACLS algorithms, insulin scales, and validated scoring systems makes bedside care efficient.

This book originated from the authors work with a growing Emergency Medicine Residency Program in the most violent county in the nation by every statistical measure, which prompted grants from the Centers for Disease Control to help curb the rural morbidity and mortality the authors encounter daily.

The authors trained at institutions ranging from Northwestern University Hospital, Wake Forest School of Medicine, and Duke University with more than 80 years combined emergency medicine experience. We also felt it was important to have a comprehensively diverse author team that includes a board certified Emergency Physician, a Physician Assistant, and a Nurse Practitioner.

We hope you will agree that this is the most efficient and utilitarian pocket text available.

Phillip M. Stephens, DHSc, PA-C
Jeffery A. Klein, MD, FACEP
Gina S. Stephens, DNP, FNP-BC

Abdominal Aortic Aneurysm 1

☐ GENERAL

Mortality rate is high in rupture—elective repair most effective management to prevent rupture[1]

Majority of the population (95%) have an aortic diameter < 3 cm[2]

- Aneurysmal is defined as > 3 cm
  - Small < 4 cm
  - Medium 4–5.5 cm
  - Large > 5.5 cm

Smoking is an important variable contributing to expansion[3]

Risk factors: advanced age—cigarette smoking—male—Caucasian—HTN—atherosclerosis—family history of AAA—Other aneurysms[4]

■ EVALUATION

Classic presentation of severe pain, pulsatile abdominal mass, & hypotension occurs in only 50% of cases[5]

- Misdiagnosis for conditions, such as renal colic, ischemic bowel, or GI hemorrhage occurs in 30% of cases[6]

Labs not specific

- CBC—ESR—U/A are useful in evaluating other causes of pain

Asymptomatic AAA may be suspected based on history or incidental finding

- Imaging to confirm, determine extent, and manage rupture risk

Symptomatic AAA: abdominal, flank or back pain—flank ecchymosis—evidence of an aortic fistula

Hemodynamically stable-abdominal CT[7]

Hemodynamically unstable-ultrasound[7]

■ MANAGEMENT

Consult surgery: Management is dependent on the diameter & presence of symptoms. Options include stenting vs graft/surgery

Unstable patients require resuscitation & emergent surgical repair

2 Abdominal Pain

GENERAL

History & physical exam sensitivity in determining etiology of abdominal pain is poor[1]
- Accuracy for more serious causes of pain is better than for benign causes[2]
- CBC can be normal in the face of serious disease such as appendicitis[3,4]
- Early appendicitis & early SBO are the two most common reasons for erroneous discharge[5]

No strict time differentiates acute from chronic. Pain less than several days is acute & unchanged for months is chronic
- Pain >few days but <a few months is subacute with a broader differential

Most common ER visit[6]
- Location is suggestive of diagnosis[7]

Red flags: age > 50 yo, weight loss, persistent vomiting, dysphagia, anemia, hematemesis, palpable abdominal mass, FHx of upper GI cancer, previously known pathology, or surgery of pathology that could recur

Consider rare causes of abdominal pain: Repeated visits for the same complaint without definite diagnosis, pain out of proportion to findings, illness appearing with nonspecific findings, immunocompromised patient (nonverbal elderly patients sometimes need more extensive evaluation)

High risk: age over 65 yo, immunocompromised, ETOH, CV disease, early pregnancy, major comorbidities, prior surgery, sudden onset, maximum pain at onset, pain then vomiting, constant pain less than 2 days: rigid abdomen, shock, guarding

DDx of life-threatening conditions: AAA, aortic dissection, mesenteric ischemia, perforation of viscus, bowel obstruction, volvulus, incarcerated hernia, splenic rupture, ectopic pregnancy, placental abruption, and myocardial infarction

EVALUATION

Studies vary depending on suspected etiology

Immediate resuscitation & surgical consult if toxic, shock, or peritoneal signs
- Bedside ultrasound helpful noting aorta, hemoperitoneum, pericardium, & IVC

In general[7]:

CBC	AAS x-ray (free air/constipation)
Chem 7	CT abd/pelvis
Hepatic panel	CT stone chaser (kidney stones)
Lipase	
HCG in women	
Blood culture × 2 if febrile or unstable	
Pelvic exam for GYN pathology: wet prep, STD cultures	

Consider RUQ ultrasound if biliary pain is suspected
Consider pelvic ultrasound if pregnant and ectopic is suspected or pelvic etiology concerns
Consider B-hydroxybutyrate if DKA is suspected
Consider retic count if sickle cell patient
Consider cardiac workup in upper abd pain with cardiac risk factors
Consider stone chaser CT if renal colic is suspected (or renal ultrasound if young or hx of multiple CTs)
Consider Strep test in children & pharyngeal findings
Consider serum lactic acid if intestinal ischemia/metabolic acidosis suspected

MANAGEMENT

Treat underlying cause
  Observation & serial exams may be necessary[6]
Multiple RCTs demonstrate early analgesia does not hinder management decisions prior to determining etiology of abdominal pain[8]
Consider Morphine (0.1 mg/kg) 4–6 mg IV in adults[9]
Elderly admit if any doubt of diagnosis
  (Cholecystitis in elderly may present with just fever and no abdominal pain. Obstruction will most likely have vomiting and abd pain)
Any discharge consideration should include comorbidities, social support, reliability, and understanding of clear return instructions

□ GENERAL

ABG is the gold standard for evaluating respiratory status & acid/base disturbances[1]

Pulse oximetry is used as an adjunct to assess trends & decrease invasive procedures[1]

Absolute contraindications for sampling:

Abnormal Allen's Test, local infection at site, severe peripheral vascular disease, or active Raynaud's syndrome[2]

Venous pH is an acceptable alternative to ABG in initial management with a high degree of correlation to arterial pH[3]

■ EVALUATION

1. Identify the primary disorder by the pH (acidosis or alkalosis)[4]
2. Differentiate respiratory & metabolic components by the pCO_2 & HCO_3
3. Assess for compensation
4. Assess for hypoxemia

Examine pH:	Normal	7.35–7.45
	Acidosis	< 7.35
	Alkalosis	> 7.45
Examine pCO_2:	Normal	35–45 (respiratory component)
	Respiratory alkalosis	< 35
	Respiratory acidosis	> 45
Examine HCO_3:	Normal	24–26 (renal component)
	Metabolic acidosis	< 24
	Metabolic alkalosis	> 26

Determine if there is compensation for the pH balance

Pulmonary & renal systems generally compensate for each to return the pH to normal

Resp Acidosis (↓pH: ↑pCO_2) HCO_3 increased = Compensation

Resp Alkalosis (↑pH: ↓pCO_2) HCO_3 decreased = Compensation
Met Acidosis (↓pH: ↓HCO_3) pCO_2 decreased = Compensation
Met Alkalosis (↑pH: ↑HCO_3) pCO_2 increased = Compensation

Examine pO_2:	Normal	80–100
	Hypoxemia	< 80

1 to 10 Rule:

In acute setting: **For every 10 units that pCO_2 rises:**

pH decreases by 0.08 (almost 1 unit)

HCO_3 increases by 1 in acidosis (pCO_2 rises) and **decreases by 2 in alkalosis** (pCO_2 falls)

Example: given a baseline pH of 7.40 & pCO_2 40

Hypoventilation, raising pCO_2 to 50: pH will decrease to 7.32

Hyperventilation, decreasing pCO_2 to 30: pH will increase to 7.48

ROME method:

Respiratory = **Opposite:**	Metabolic = **Equal:**
pH ↑: pCO_2 ↓ (alkalosis)	pH ↑: HCO_3 ↑ (alkalosis)
pH ↓: pCO_2 ↑ (acidosis)	pH ↓: HCO_3 ↓ (acidosis)

Dialysis/CRF pts will have low HCO_3 values[5]
Chronic COPD can have HCO_3 of 42 or even higher & baseline pCO_2 of 100+[6]

MANAGEMENT

Treat underlying cause

Arterial Blood Gas Interpretation Reference			
Normal range: pH 7.35–7.45, $PaCO_2$ 35–45 mm Hg, PaO_2 80–100 mm Hg, HCO_3 22–26 mEg/L			
Disorder	**pH**	**Primary disturbance**	**Compensation**
Respiratory acidosis	↓	↑ PCO_2	↑ HCO_3
Respiratory alkalosis	↑	↓ PCO_2	↓ HCO_3
Metabolic acidosis	↓	↓ HCO_3	↓ PCO_2
Metabolic alkalosis	↑	↑ HCO_3	↑ PCO_2

☐ GENERAL

- Acetaminophen (APAP) is the most common cause of liver failure from a single ingestion or repeated supratherapeutic ingestions[1]
  - Occurs from intentional harm (single dose) or therapeutic attempts typically with drugs containing APAP[2]
- Hepatotoxicity potential[3]:
  - Single ingestion dose > or = 200 mg/kg or 10 g (whichever is less) in < 8-hour period
  - Repeated ingestion in age > 6 yo
    - ≥ 200 mg/kg or 10 g (whichever is less) < 24-hour period
    - ≥ 150 mg/kg or 6 g/d (whichever is less) < 48-hour period
    - ≥ 100 mg/kg/d or 4 g/d if risk factors (pregnant, chronic ETOH, fasting, isoniazid use)
  - Repeated ingestion age < 6 yo
    - ≥ 200 mg/kg within 24-hour period
    - ≥ 150 mg/kg/d within 48-hour period
    - ≥ 100 mg/kg/d within 72-hour period
- No specific early findings—OD presents in 4 phases after ingestion[3]

Phase 1 (first 24 hours):	Asymptomatic. May have nonspecific symptoms (nausea, diaphoresis, lethargy, malaise)
Phase 2 (24–72 hours):	Symptoms may improve or disappear. Prolonged prothrombin time and increased transaminases
	Increased hepatotoxicity risk if care sought > 24 hours post ingestion
Phase 3 (72–96 hours):	Liver injury peaks. Symptoms reappear or worsen
	May have malaise, jaundice, renal failure CNS symptoms such as confusion
Phase 4 (96–14 days):	Patient progresses to death by multiorgan failure or recovers within 3 months

4 Acetaminophen OD

EVALUATION

Attempt to determine ingestion dose & if in combination with other drugs along with timing & reason for ingestion
- Young adults typically have high APAP exposures that do not contain opioids[4]
- Adults strike toxic from chronic exposure are typically from lower doses strike with opioids[4]

Assess for other drugs that may increase hepatotoxicity[1]
- Rifampin, Isoniazid, Phenobarbital, Statins, Fibrates, NSAIDs

If time of ingestion is known: consult Rumack–Matthew nomogram to assess toxicity potential[5]
- Nomogram not indicated for:
  - Unknown ingestion time
  - Repeated supratherapeutic ingestion
  - > 24 hours since acute single ingestion

If time is unknown or repeated supratherapeutic ingestions—use last ingestion free period as guide[5]

Labs[3,6]: APAP level 4 hours post ingestion (Rumack–Matthew nomogram guides treatment)
- Chemistries and hepatic panel (for ALT, AST, alkaline phosphatase, bilirubin)
- PT/INR, PTT
- CBC (platelet count, Hgb)
- ABG for arterial pH
- Serum amylase
- Lactate levels

MANAGEMENT

See also Chapter 76

Contact Poison Control Center (National 800-222-1222)
- Children age < 7 yo safe for home monitoring if ingestion < 200 mg/kg[7]

Consider activated charcoal (AC) if < 4 hours post ingestion[3,8]
- (Contraindications include: patients not able to protect airway, vomiting, co-ingestion of a corrosive or proconvulsant)[3,8,9]

Some recommendations are to administer if < 1–2 hours or later if massive ingestion[3]

No findings that AC interferes significantly with N-acetylcysteine (NAC)[3,10]
1 g/kg (max dose 50 g)
Induced emesis & gastric lavage less effective and not recommended[11]
NAC indications[3,12]
(ideally < 8 hours: antidote to hepatotoxic effects of metabolites—will not affect APAP levels)[8]
- 4-hour APAP above Rumack–Matthew nomogram treatment line
- Single ingestion > 150 mg/kg (7.5 g total dose regardless of weight)
  If APAP level will not be available > 8 hours from ingestion time
- Unknown time of ingestion with APAP concentration > 10 mcg/mL
- APAP ingestion and any evidence of liver injury (specifically if delayed presentation > 24 hours post ingestion)
  Manage in consultation with poison control center or a toxicologist

IV adult load 150 mg/kg in 200 mL diluent over 1 hour—followed by 50 mg/kg in 500 mL diluent over 4 hours—followed by 100 mg/kg in 1000 mL diluent over 16 hours[3]
Po load dose 140 mg/kg—followed by 70 mg/kg po every 4 hours for 18 total doses[3,13]
There are 20-hour IV protocols and 72-hour po protocols—both IV & po seem to have similar effectiveness[14]
IV favored if: vomiting—hepatic failure present—patients refusing po—contraindications to po (pancreatitis, bowel obstruction, or ileus)
NAC treatment is the same in pregnant patients (typically IV due to vomiting risk)[15]

Acetaminophen OD

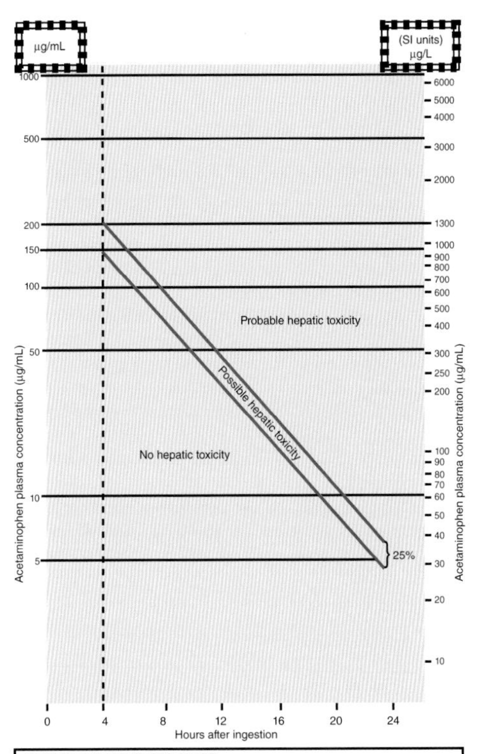

CAUTION FOR USE OF THIS CHART

1. The time coordinates refer to time of ingestion.
2. Serum levels drawn before 4 hours may not represent peak levels.
3. The graph should be used only in relation to a single acute ingestion.
4. The lower solid line is 25% below the standard nomogram and is included to allow for possible errors in acetaminophen plasma assays and estimated time from ingestion of an overdose.

VF/PULSELESS VT

Start CPR (30 compressions: 2 respirations): oxygen
Attach defibrillator—analyze rhythm (rate: fast vs slow—QRS: wide vs narrow—rhythm: regular vs irregular)
Shockable VF/pulseless VT = 360 J (monophasic), 200 J (biphasic)
If not shockable go to asystole/PEA algorithm
No pulse = CPR 2 minutes: push hard/fast (IV access)
After 2 minutes: shockable VF/pulseless VT = 360 J (monophasic)
Epi 1 mg IV/IO every 3–5 minutes
Consider advanced airway
CPR 2 minutes
Shockable VF/pulseless VT = 360 J (monophasic), 200 J (biphasic)
Amiodarone IV/IO 300 mg IV bolus
Second dose 150 mg IV bolus

Consider reversible causes:

Hypovolemia	Tension pneumothorax	Hypothermia
Hypoxia	Tamponade (cardiac)	
Hydrogen ion (acidosis)	Toxins	
Hypo or hyperkalemia	Thrombosis: pulmonary or cardiac	

ASYSTOLE/PEA

No shockable VT/pulseless VT[1]
CPR 2 minutes = IV Access
Epi 1 mg IV/IO every 3–5 minutes
Treat reversible causes

BRADYCARDIA WITH A PULSE

HR < 50 (however in clinical practice usually HR ≤ 40 should raise your awareness that patient needs to be seen quickly)
Maintain airway: O_2 if hypoxemic

Monitor: IV access: ECG: if *stable* continue to monitor
Assess stability
  Hypotension?
  Acute mental status changes?
  Shock?
  Chest pain?
  Heart failure?

UNSTABLE BRADYCARDIA

Atropine IV 0.5 mg bolus repeat every 3–5 min (max 3 mg)
If ineffective: transcutaneous pacing
or
Dopamine infusion 2–20 mcg/kg/min
or
Epi infusion 2–10 mcg/min

TACHYCARDIA

HR > 150
Treat underlying cause: O_2 if hypoxemic: monitor
Synchronized cardioversion if unstable (ie, hypotension, acute mental status changes, shock, chest pain, heart failure)
If stable: wide complex
  Consider adenosine only if regular monomorphic
  Consider antiarrhythmic infusion—procainamide
  Consider expert consultation
If stable: narrow complex
  Vagal maneuvers
  Adenosine (if regular)
  β-blocker or calcium channel blocker (monitor blood pressure closely with calcium channel blocker)
  Consider expert consult

Adult Cardiac Arrest Algorithm—2015 Update

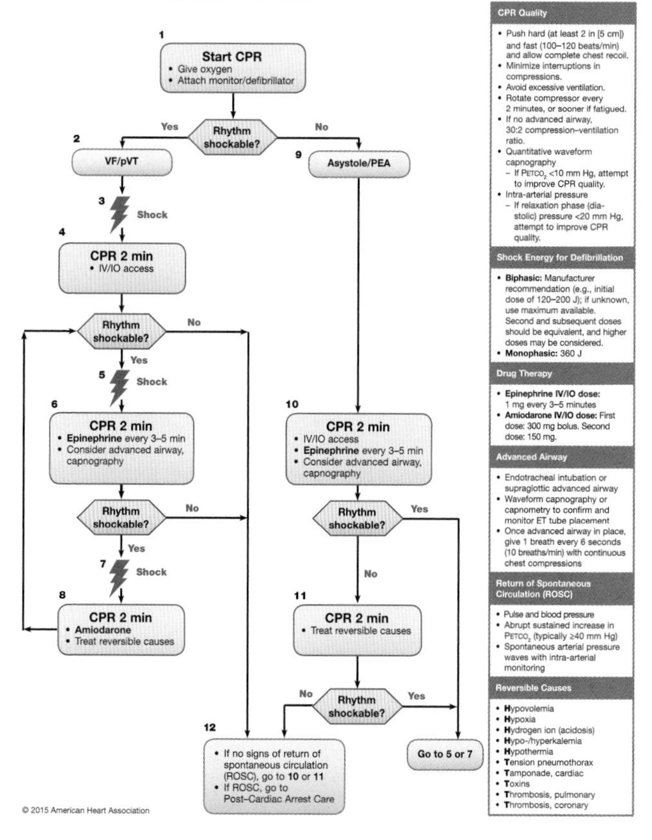

Adult Tachycardia Algorithm with a Pulse Algorithm

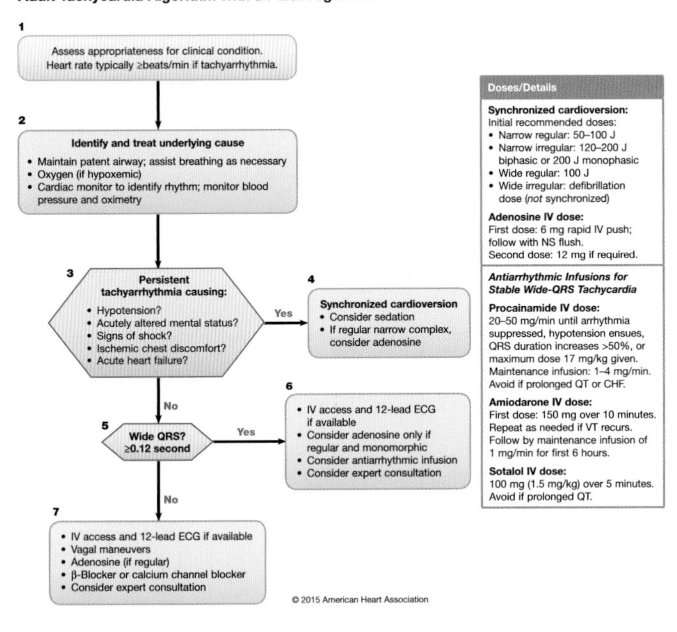

Adult Bradycardia with a Pulse Algorithm

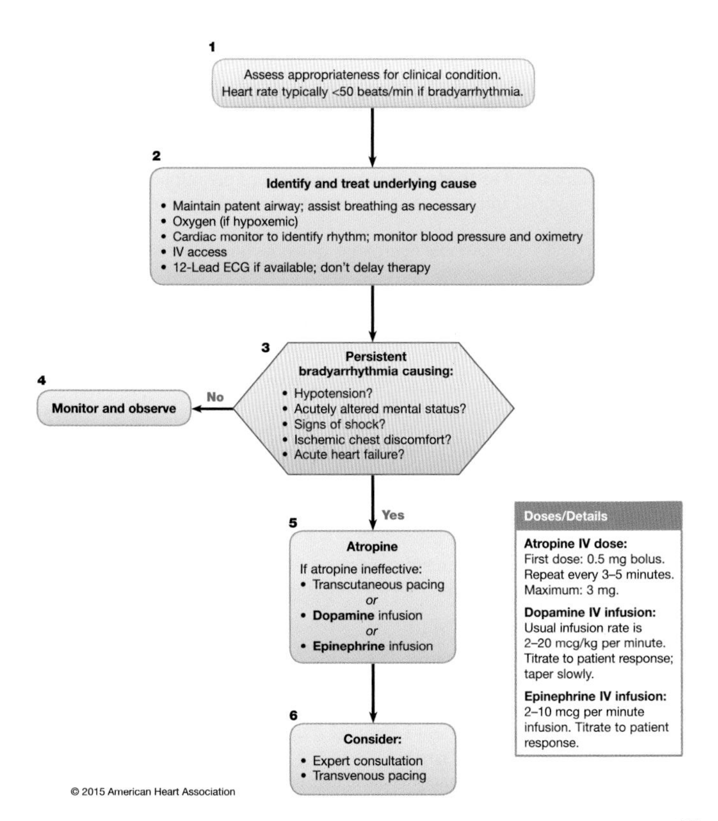

6 ACLS General

☐ GENERAL

ACLS Guidelines are continually reviewed & formally released every 5 years
Excellent CPR (push hard, push fast) with few interruptions & early defibrillation of shockable rhythms are the foundation of recommendations[1]
  Every effort should be made to not interrupt CPR (circulation-airway-breathing: CAB)
Arrest patients are often over ventilated compromising cardiac output[2]
  No advanced airway—30 : 2 compression to ventilation ratio
  Advanced airway—8 to 10 asynchronous ventilations per minute
Advanced airways (ET intubation) has no advantage over bag valve mask (BVM) ventilation[3]
  Rate of survival with favorable neurologic outcome higher with BVM in a prospective study[3]
  Studies support a basic approach to airway management is acceptable though some studies are observational with limitations

■ EVALUATION

Start CPR
Administer oxygen
Attach monitor/defibrillator
Analyze rhythm

■ MANAGEMENT

Follow ACLS guidelines
Decision to discontinue resuscitation efforts
  Death in hospital is more likely if all 4 conditions are present[4]:
1. Patients age > 75 yo
2. Unwitnessed arrest
3. Resuscitation > 10 minutes
4. Initial cardiac rhythm not VT or V-fib

  Criteria predictive of less chance of survival in out-of-hospital arrest[5]:
1. Out-of-hospital arrest not witnessed
2. Non-shockable initial rhythm
3. No spontaneous circulation before third dose of epinephrine

Acute Coronary Syndrome

☐ GENERAL

Risk factors:
- Prior MI—CAD—sedentary lifestyle—obesity—tobacco use—HTN—HLD—DM
- Family Hx (CV event < 55-yo men/< 65-yo women)—chronic kidney disease—vascular disease[1,2]
- Cocaine use greatly increases MI risk within first 60 minutes of usage[3]
- Regular cocaine use associated with increased nonfatal risk[3]

Pressure type retrosternal area discomfort at rest or with minimal exertion[3]

Dyspnea[3]

■ EVALUATION

Assess risk of acute ischemic pain
- Risk factors—pain characteristics—past medical Hx—family Hx—social Hx[3]
- Clinical features alone are insufficient for diagnosis and have limited role[3,4]

Assess ASA use & other medications
- ASA reduces MI risk[3]
- Sildenafil in conjunction with nitrate administration contraindicated due to possible refractory hypotension[3]

Physical exam: assess for etiology of pain and/or heart failure[3]

Consider: aortic aneurysm, PE, pneumothorax, esophageal rupture, perforated ulcer, pericarditis, cardiac tamponade, pleuritis

Testing:
- ECG (on arrival, repeat at 15–30 minute intervals if non-diagnostic & pt remains symptomatic)[5]
- Continuous ECG monitoring
- Troponin (elevations noted 3–6 hours after symptom onset)

Tests to identify comorbidities & guide mgt[6]:
- Portable CXR
- CBC
- Chemistry panel (BMP–electrolytes)
- PT, PTT
- Magnesium

Immediate cardiac cath in non-ST elevation ACS with refractory angina, hemodynamic, or electrical instability[6]

Immediate cardiac cath with percutaneous coronary intervention (PCI) if available in ST elevation[7]

MANAGEMENT

Antiplatelet therapy: ASA 162–365 mg (chewed)[6]
Nitroglycerin: 0.3–0.4 mg sublingually q 5 min up to 3 doses
Followed by IV nitrates in persistent pain, HTN or heart failure (avoid for patients who are hypotensive or have taken a phosphodiesterase inhibitor med for erectile dysfunction in previous 24 hours)
Oxygen: only if sats < 94%[8,9]
Morphine: reasonable for pain
β-blocker: po first 24 hours unless contraindicated
(no heart failure, low output state or risk of cardiogenic shock that increases with age > 70 yo, systolic BP < 120, tachy > 110, HR < 60) or relative contraindications such as heart block or asthma
No randomized controlled trials specifically addressing benefit in non-ST elevation ACS (benefits known in MI & there are no deleterious effect on NSTEMI)
Metoprolol (EF > 40%): preferred agent as it is cardioselective
Unstable angina: 2.5–5 mg IV q 5 min up to total 15 mg then 25–50 mg PO 15 minutes later
HTN: 25–100 mg PO qd
Carvedilol (EF < 40%):
HTN: 6.25 mg PO BID (may increase q 12 weeks 12.5 mg PO BID then 25 mg PO bid)
CHF: start 3.125 mg PO BID (may increase q 2 weeks to 6.25 mg PO BID, then 12.5 mg BID then 25 mg BID)
Esmolol:
Difficult rate control (dissection/A-fib/A-flutter: Load 500 mcg/kg IV over 1 minute—then
50 mcg/kg/min—may increase maintenance dose by 50 mcg/kg/min q 4 min prn—max: 300 mcg/kg/min
Labetelol (HTN drug of choice):
HTN emergency: start 10–20 mg IV × 1—then 40–80 mg IV q 10 min-max: 300 mg/total dose or IV infusion 0.5–2 mg/min

Calcium channel blockers: in patients with contraindications to β-blockers and ongoing ischemia unless significant LV dysfunction, increased cardiogenic shock risk, PR interval > .024 seconds, or heart block without a pacemaker
- Cardizem for A-fib rate control:
- A-fib: 0.2 mg/kg IV × 1 (**20 mg adult**) over 2 minutes
  - May repeat at 0.35 mg/kg (25 mg adult) IV × 1 after 15 minutes
  - May follow with 5–15 mg/h IV infusion for < 24 hours for ventricular rate control

Ace inhibitor/statins: Recommended for early hospital care but not IV within first 24 hours due to hypotension risk
- Recovery care from the MI not typical for ER to initiate

Anticoagulation:
- Heparin 50–60 units/kg IV (max 4000 units)—then 12 units/kg/h infusion (max 1000 units/h) with or without PCI intervention potential
- Enoxaparin Sodium 1 mg/kg SQ with ASA (unstable angina, non-Q-wave MI—if no PCI intervention)
  - Antiplatelet agents
    - Prasugrel 60 mg PO load then 10 mg daily with ASA
    - Clopidogrel 300 mg PO load then 75 mg daily with ASA
    - Ticagrelor 180 mg PO load then 90 mg BID

Electrolytes (magnesium/potassium)[10]:
- No randomized controlled trials noting benefit though cohort studies demonstrate lowest mortality with K^+ 3.5 to < 4.5 mEq/L

Arrhythmia management:
- Amiodarone
  - Pulseless VT/VF: 300 mg rapid IV bolus (follow current ACLS guidelines)
  - Stable VT: 150 mg IV over 10 minutes, then 1 mg/min for 6 hours
  - Prevention of ventricular arrhythmias: 800–1600 mg daily
- Procainamide is an alternative: 20 mg/min until arrhythmia terminates, hypotension, QRS prolongation > 50% or a total of 1.2 g given to an adult patient

Pressor agents:
- Dopamine: start 5 mcg/kg/min. Increase PRN in 5–10 mcg/kg/min increments at 10-minute intervals. Max 50 mcg/kg/min

Risk stratification:

HEART Score Risk Stratification

	Hx	Highly suspicious	2
		Moderately suspicious	1
		Slightly suspicious	0
	ECG	Significant ST-Depression	2
		Nonspecific	1
		Normal	0
	Age	> or = 65	2
		45–65	1
		< or = 45	0
	Risk factors	> or = 3	2
		1 or 2	1
		None	0
	Troponin	> or = 3 × normal	2
		1–3 × normal	1
		< or = normal	0
Score 1–2		Risk 1.6%	Recommends discharge
Score 4–6		Risk 13%	Observation vs Admit & repeat ECG
Score 7–10		Risk 50%	Admit

NORMAL LBBB	SGARBOSSA – ISCHEMIA
V1 DEEP S in V1	CONCORDANT ST DEPRESSION ≥ 1 mm in V1, V2, or V3
V1 QRS > 120 ms	EXCESSIVELY DISCORDANT ELEVATION ≥ 5 mm or ST ELEVATION/S WAVE ≥ 0.25 mm
V6 BROAD R WAVE, MAY HAVE "M" NOTCHING IN I, aVL, V5, V6	CONCORDANT ST ELEVATION ≥ 1 mm

Acute Coronary Syndrome

Composition of the HEART Score for Chest Pain Patients in the Emergency Room

HEART Score for Chest Pain Patients		Score
History	Highly suspicious	2
	Moderately suspicious	1
	Slightly suspicious	0
ECG	Significant ST depression	2
	Nonspecific repolarisation disturbance	1
	Normal	0
Age	≥ 65 yo	2
	45-65 yo	1
	< 45 yo	0
Risk factors	≥ 3 risk factors or history of atherosclerotic disease	2
	1 or 2 risk factors	1
	No risk factors known	0
Troponin	> 2 × normal limit	2
	1-2 × normal limit	1
	≤normal limit	0

Score 1-2	Risk 1.6%	Study Rec Discharge	**Total** _____
Score 4-6	Risk 13%	Obs admit & X-ECG	
Score 7-10	Risk 50%	Admit	

□ GENERAL

< 4–6 weeks = acute
> 6 weeks to 3 months = subacute/chronic
Early recognition of serious etiologies (Cauda equina/SEA) of back pain improve outcome[1]
Red flag: underlying disease: age > 50 yo, cancer, weight loss, > 1-month pain, nighttime pain, unresponsive to previous tx[2]
(drug use, bacterial infection, and fever increase spinal infection risk)
Red flag: Cauda equina syndrome (surgical emergency = decompression needed)
Progressive motor or sensory deficit
Leg weakness
Saddle anesthesia
Difficulty urinating
Fecal incontinence
(bowel & bladder dysfunction late finding present in half of the patients)[3]
Red flag: Spinal epidural abscess (SEA). Classic triad (present in a small proportion of patients)[4]
Fever
Focal spinous process pain
Neurodeficits (sensory/motor)
Be suspicious of sequence for SEA[5]:
Severe focal back pain, then nerve root pain (shooting), then motor weakness (sensory, bowel/bladder dysfunction), then paralysis (predisposing factors: recent spinal surgery, IV drug use, recent tattoo, immunocompromised, DM)

■ EVALUATION

Acute low back pain requires no lab testing in most patients
Progressive neurodeficits: urgent or emergent MRI (suspected SEA or cancer patients image entire spine)
Suspected SEA: ESR/CRP to assess the feasibility of MRI[6,7]
ESR (and CRP) has good sensitivity to differentiate need for imaging[8]
Consider U/A, CBC, blood culture depending on the presentation
CSF is generally not evaluated

Imaging in nonspecific LBP without associated symptoms (SEA/Cauda equina/ malignancy) not shown to improve outcomes[9]
Most LBP < 4 weeks duration does not require imaging if no serious associated symptoms[10]
Waddell sign for nonorganic pain:
  Overreaction during exam
  Superficial or widespread tenderness
  Inconsistent distracted straight leg raise (seated/supine)
  Unexplained neurologic deficits
  Simulated axial load (pressing on top of head) elicits pain[11]
Other distraction tests such as "Heel Tap Test" may demonstrate nonorganic evidence of pain for secondary gain[12]

Considerations for imaging[13]:

Age < 20 or > 50 yo	Significant trauma
Pain unrelenting, nonmechanical, or thoracic	Penetrating wound
Unexplained weight loss	Spine deformity
Widespread neuro symptoms	Nerve root involvement
Fever or toxic appearance	Immunocompromised (steroids, HIV, cancer)

MANAGEMENT

Bedrest not generally recommended for acute LBP. Remaining somewhat active is preferred[14]
NSAIDs/muscle relaxants
Opioids considered if used judiciously for severe or debilitating pain
Assess patient narcotic usage via the State Narcotic Database before prescribing narcotics

☐ GENERAL

Tolerance & dependence occurs with chronic ETOH use[1]
- Biologic tolerance may result in withdrawal symptoms even with significant ETOH levels[2]

Minor withdrawal (6–36 hours after last ingestion): headache, mild anxiety, tremors, palpitations, normal mental status[2]

Seizures (6–48 hours after last ingestion): tonic-clonic, short postictal, status epilepticus rare[2]

ETOH hallucinosis (12–48 hours after last ingestion): visual or auditory hallucinations, orientation intact, vital signs normal[2]

Delirium tremens (48–96 hours after last ingestion): delirium, agitation, hypertension, tachycardia, diaphoresis, fever[2]

Withdrawal seizures can occur as early as 2 hours post ingestion[3]
- Role of anticonvulsants unclear—left untreated can progress to delirium tremens in 1/3 of patients[3]

■ EVALUATION

History of drinking & last ingestion
- Chronicity & history of withdrawal symptoms

Physical exam for evidence of withdrawal spectrum
- Varying agitation—mild tachycardia—mild tremors—normal mental status
- Then hallucinations are possible without delirium
- Then seizures though this may be the presenting symptom (single without prolonged postictal phase)
- DTs are the most severe complication

Consider Wernicke's encephalopathy (thiamine deficiency) if[4]:
- Nystagmus—altered mental status—cranial nerve abnormalities—gait disturbance

DT risk factors[5]
- History of sustained drinking
- History of DTs
- Age > 30 yo
- Withdrawal symptoms in presence of elevated ETOH
- The presence of concurrent illness
- Prolonged period since last drink but with withdrawal symptoms

Labs (no specific test is diagnostic for withdrawal)[6]:
- Glucose immediately
- CBC
- Chemistries (electrolytes, lipase, & liver functions: Consider ammonia level)
- Magnesium/phosphate
- ETOH level (the presence of ETOH does not exclude withdrawal risk)
- Lactate level (evaluate unexplained anion gap metabolic acidosis)
- Beta-hydroxybutyrate (if ETOH ketoacidosis suspected)
- U/A with drug testing (HCG females)
- CT head if mental status changes
- CXR for pulmonary symptoms
- Consider: ECG, troponin in chest pain, and/or cardiac history or ECG age > 50 yo
  - Lumbar puncture for mental status changes
  - TSH: hyperthyroidism suspected (typically a longer course of symptoms)

Consider validated assessment scales to monitor severity such as:
- Clinical Institute Withdrawal Assessment for Alcohol (CIWA-Ar)

Exclude comorbid illness

■ MANAGEMENT

IVFs with Thiamine 100 mg IV before glucose[7]
- Magnesium sulfate has not been shown to improve withdrawal[8]
- Magnesium sulfate is appropriate if hypomagnesemic[8]
- Traditional "Banana Bags" with Thiamine, Folate, vitamins in 5% Dextrose are not well studied & may not meet needs

Nutritional support (multivitamins)

Frequent vital sign monitoring

Benzodiazepine first-line therapy[9-11]
- Lorazepam 2 mg IV or IM can be repeated every 30 minutes
  - If given too frequently can cause sedative stacking
- Diazepam 10–20 mg IV q 5–10 min until effect
  - Caution in chronic liver failure, which prolongs half-life
- Chlordiazepoxide 25–100 mg po q 1 h first 2–3 hours

Phenytoin is ineffective[12]

Refractory DTs not clearly defined

- Typically if lorazepam 10 mg or diazepam 50 mg is required to control in 1st hour[13]
  - or lorazepam 40 mg (diazepam 200 mg) first 3 hours[13]
- Add phenobarbital 130–260 mg IV q 15–20 min until controlled[13]
  - or Phenobarbital 65–130 mg IV over 5 minutes initially—wait 40 minutes before redosing
- Single phenobarbital regimens (10 mg/kg in 100 mL NS) have been investigated[14]

Consider propofol (opens chloride channels)[15]

- Intubation typically needed if phenobarbital & propofol are needed

Antipsychotics may be used if psychiatric disorders coexist—use with caution

- Avoid haloperidol as it lowers seizure threshold[16]

CIWA scores > 15 or DT symptoms (disorientation, fever, diaphoresis, tachycardia, hypertension): admit

CIWA scores 8–15 without DT symptoms or seizures may qualify for ambulatory detoxification if also[17]:

- Able to take po meds
- Reliable social support to assist patient (3–5 days) & monitor
- Medical conditions stable
- Able to commit to daily medical visits
- Not psychotic, suicidal, or cognitively impaired
- Not pregnant
- No concomitant drug abuse that may exacerbate withdrawal
- No history of DT or withdrawal symptoms
- Relative contraindications for ambulatory setting: age > 60 yo, end-organ damage evidence (renal insufficiency, cirrhosis)

10 Angioedema

☐ GENERAL

Self-limited sudden localized tissue swelling due to leakage of plasma into the interstitial space[1]
- May be accompanied by urticaria (histaminergic)[1]
- Generally affects loose connective tissue (face, lips, extremities, genitalia, bowel wall)
- Rapid onset—not involving gravity dependent areas as in chronic edema

Histaminergic more common[1]
- Idiopathic—allergic—drug induced
  - May be accompanied by urticaria
  - Generally responds to antihistamines (ie, allergy induced)

Nonhistaminergic angioedema[1,2]
- No urticaria or allergic symptoms[2]
- Slower to develop (24–36 hours)—more prolonged course
- Relationship to a trigger, less striking (ie, ACE inhibitor induced may occur after weeks or years of use)
- May involve the bradykinin pathway & not respond to antihistamines

Anaphylaxis is angioedema associated with hypotension & respiratory compromise[1]

■ EVALUATION

Assess airway

Identify possible causes (ACE inhibitors, NSAIDs, insect stings)

Symptoms of allergic reaction (mast cell activation-urticaria, pruritus, throat tightening) narrows the cause to ingestions or exposures[1,3]

Symptoms without urticaria and unresponsive to antihistamines may be bradykinin mediated (ACE inhibitor, acquired C1 inhibitor deficiency)[1]

Generally a clinical diagnosis—routine labs in acute setting may not be helpful[1]
- Chronic or unclear trigger consider:
  - CBC
  - Chemistry
  - CRP or ESR (may be elevated during infection process or ACE inhibitor induced)[4]

Complement protein C4
Decreased C4 suggests hereditary or acquired C1 inhibitor deficiency
TSH
Fiberoptic laryngoscopy if available to assess airway angioedema[1]
CT abdomen/pelvis if there is suspicion of bowel wall involvement (ACE inhibitor induced—angioedema associated with abdominal pain usually suggests hereditary angioedema)[5,6]
Ascites—small bowel wall thickening—straightening

■ MANAGEMENT

Secure airway if compromised (anaphylaxis)[7]
Epinephrine (1 mg/mL) 0.3–0.5 IM can repeat every 5–15 minutes
Can give IV infusion if not responding (0.1 mcg/kg/min)
IVF
Oxygen
Albuterol neb
Vasopressors
Glucagon (patients taking β-blockers may not respond to epinephrine) (1–5 mg IV over 5 minutes—then infusion 5–15 mcg/min)
Allergic (urticaria): stop cause
H1 antihistamines (diphenhydramine 25–50 mg IV)
Glucocorticoid (methylprednisolone 125 mg IV—prednisone 20–40 mg po daily over 5–7 days)
Epinephrine (0.3–0.5 mg IM); (0.01 mg/kg—max 0.5 mg per single dose). Can repeat in 5–15 minutes
H2 antihistamine (ranitidine 50 mg IV)
Nonhistaminergic: known hereditary or acquired angioedema
C1 inhibitor concentrate
Nonhistaminergic: ACE inhibitor mediated—stop med
Supportive care
Observe patients who do not require admission for improvement

11 Ankle/Foot/Knee

OTTAWA ANKLE/FOOT

Applied to adult patients with pain due to trauma (blunt, twist, fall, direct blow)[1]

Does not apply to patients < 18 yo, isolated skin injury, injury > 10 days, intoxication, head injury, multiple painful injuries, or diminished sensation due to neuro deficit

Ankle x-ray only required if pain at the malleolar area AND

- Bone tenderness at posterior edge or tip of
- Lateral OR
- Medial malleolus OR
- Inability to bear weight both immediately and in ER

Foot x-ray only required if the pain is in midfoot AND/OR

- Tenderness at the fifth metatarsal base or navicular bone OR
- Inability to bear weight both immediately and in ER

OTTAWA KNEE

X-ray acute knee injury if[2]

- > 55 yo
- Tenderness in the fibula head
- Isolated patella tenderness
- Inability to flex knee to 90°
- Inability to bear weight immediately or in ER
  - (defined as 4 steps with the ability to transfer weight twice to each LE regardless of limping)

Exclusion criteria:

< 18 yo	altered LOC
Isolated skin injury	paraplegia
Injury > 7 days	multiple injury
Recent injury being reevaluated	

PITTSBURGH KNEE

Appears more specific than Ottawa rules with no sensitivity loss[3]

X-ray knee injury if

- Age < 12 yo or > 50 yo in fall or direct force injury
- Age 12–50 yo in fall & unable to walk 4 weight-bearing steps in ER

Exclusion criteria:

- Injuries > 6 days old
- Superficial abrasions & lacerations only
- Previous knee surgeries same knee
- Reassessment of same injury (repeat visit)

Outside of these rules do not forget to evaluate the ankle for Achilles tendon injury with the Thompson test (lay patient prone, have pt relax the leg while you hold it, and squeeze the calf to eval for plantar flexion)

For the knee eval for a patellar tendon injury (ie, see if the patient can extend the knee)

12 Anxiety Disorder

☐ GENERAL

Difficult to control worry/anxiety more days than not for at least 6 months (generalized anxiety disorder)[1]

Typical timing pattern:

- 10–15 minutes prior to stress event (perception trigger) = **Panic disorder**
- 10–15 minutes prior to stress event (specific trigger: spider, blood) = **Phobia**
- Within days of traumatic event = **Acute stress disorder**
- One month or more after traumatic event = **PTSD**
- All the time = **Generalized anxiety disorder**

■ EVALUATION

Inquire about drug use[2]

Consider depression, bipolar, psychosis, or withdrawal from ETOH, benzodiazepines, sedative hypnotics, opiates

Consider hyperthyroidism, cardiopulmonary disorders, traumatic brain injury, seizure, pheochromocytoma[3]

Ensure patient is not having suicidal or homicidal ideations

Scoring systems helpful: GAD-7 and Hamilton (HAM-A)[4,5]

■ MANAGEMENT

General emergency meds

- Lorazepam 1–2 mg IV/IM[6]
- Hydroxyzine 50–100 mg PO QID[7]
- Olanzapine 5–10 mg IM (agitation, bipolar)[8]
- Haloperidol 2–5 mg IM (agitation, schizophrenia), may readminister q 60 min if necessary[9]

Typical combination: Ativan 1 mg and Zyprexa 10 mg (recommendation is to not give more than 1 mg of Lorazepam in combination with Zyprexa)

SSRIs: first-line panic disorders

- Citalopram—start 10 mg/d and titrate to 20–40 mg/d
- Sertraline—start 25 mg/d and titrate to 100–200 mg/d

Refer to a mental health professional

Admit[10]
- Acute suicidal ideations
- Substance abuse requiring detox
- Severe panic disorder when outpatient ineffective or impractical

Ketamine has been studied & trending as a treatment for severe agitation (1 mg/kg IV or 3 mg/kg IM)[11]

13 Asthma

☐ GENERAL

Inflammation of airway resulting in a hyper response & airflow limitation[1]
Peak flow measurements assess severity[2]
  Peak flow < 50% of baseline is indicative of a severe attack
Mortality risk factors include: previous asthma admissions— > 3 ER visits annually—recent steroid administration— > 1 MDI canister use a month—intubation history—illicit drug use—comorbidities
Symptoms: cough, wheezing, chest tightness, dyspnea

■ EVALUATION

The exam may be normal—wheezing increases the chance that asthma is present, but may be absent[1]
  Diagnosis based on history, physical, and spirometry[1]
Peak expiratory flow rate (PEFR)
  More useful as a monitoring tool rather than diagnostics[1]
Pulse oximetry
CXR is not required unless there is suspicion of an underlying condition such as a pneumothorax[1]
CBC may show mild leukocytosis or eosinophilia
Tachypnea, tachycardia, accessory muscle use, & breathlessness indicate severe airflow obstruction but are not sensitive indicators of a severe attack as up to 50% of severe disease will not have these abnormalities[3,4]

■ MANAGEMENT

Self-care plans[3]:
  Short-acting beta agonist (SABA) albuterol by MDI or nebulized treatment
  Good response: no wheezing or dyspnea & PEF > 80% predicted
    Follow-up routinely
    Continue SABA
    Consider a short steroid course (Prednisone 40 mg PO daily x3 days burst dose)
  Incomplete response: persistent wheezing & dyspnea, & PEF 50–79% predicted
    Add po systemic steroid course (consider 12-day tapering dose)
    Continue SABA
    Monitor closely

Poor response: marked wheezing & dyspnea, & PEF < 50%
Add po systemic steroid
Repeat SABA
May require urgent intervention
Patients presenting need assessment for a response from their self-care plan
General guide: peak flow < 200 L/min is severe obstruction or < 50% baseline for that patient[4]
Hypercapnia rare if peak flow > 25% normal or > 200 L/min[5]
This makes ABGs less necessary unless dyspnea is persistent despite bronchodilator therapy
Oxygen (particularly SpO_2 < 92%)[6]
Goal > 92%/> 95% pregnancy
Albuterol nebulization q 20 mins 3 doses
Anticholinergic nebulization
Ipratropium can be used in addition to albuterol[1]
Systemic glucocorticoids[1]
Optimal dose unknown—po & IV equally efficacious[7]
Magnesium sulfate 2 g infused over 20 minutes recommended for life-threatening cases
Severe—peak flow < 40% baseline[1]
Anesthetic agents (IV ketamine, inhaled halothane) have case reports of efficacy, mechanism unclear, case reports of adverse outcomes, & no consistent RCTs[8]
Helium-oxygen has theoretical benefit
Empiric antimicrobials not recommended[9]
Discharge patients with good response to treatment with PEF > 80%[1]
Decisions are case by case, dependent on the patient's knowledge of disease
Refer to current guidelines for meds: SABA, steroids
Intubation is a clinical decision
Admit:
Impending respiratory failure
Worsening symptoms despite treatment
Incomplete response after 1–3 hours observation PEF 60-80% predicted
Admission decision on a case-by-case basis

14 Backboard Clearance

□ GENERAL

Suspected spinal injuries should be immobilized (c-collar, backboard, lat supports) prior to ER arrival if there is no prehospital method for spinal clearance[1]
- No high-quality evidence exists that backboards prevent spinal injury or improve outcomes[2]
- Backboard practice causes anxiety and can aggravate underlying injuries. Vomiting, bleeding, and swelling are common problems on backboards. Breathing can be restricted[3]
- Allowing patients to remain on backboards for prolonged periods increases the risk of pressure ulcers & discomfort[4]
- Due to discomfort, complications, & tissue breakdown—rapid removal (**within 20–30 minutes**) from the backboard, if possible, is recommended[5]
- No documented case of worsening c-spine injury from intubation procedure[6]

■ EVALUATION

Refer **Nexus & Canadian C-spine rules** given below for removal, which is best accomplished during logroll portion of the exam

Consistent with Nexus/Canadian C-spine rule—if any of the following are present, c-spine cannot be cleared[7]
- **N**euro deficit
- **S**pinal tenderness (midline)
- **A**ltered mental status
- **I**ntoxication
- **D**istracting injury

Plain C-spine film has low sensitivity missing > 50% of clinically significant c-spine injuries[7]

CT superior study if high-risk features cause suspicion for injury—plain film adds little additional info—though justifying the higher radiation in low-risk injury is difficult[8]

MANAGEMENT

No standard approach to backboard clearance has been defined

Clear backboard patients from the board as early as feasible using Nexus/Canadian C-spine rules

Patients with reduced consciousness have a higher prevalence of c-spine injury & spinal clearance is less clear-cut as most are cleared with imaging[9,10]

15 Bell's Palsy

☐ GENERAL

Usually unilateral facial paralysis

Secondary causes include: Lyme disease, mononucleosis, Ramsay Hunt syndrome (zoster of geniculate ganglion), HIV, otitis media, parotid tumors[1]

Guillain-Barre syndrome (bilateral more likely in GBS, Lyme, myasthenia gravis, sarcoidosis)[1]

CVA mimicking Bell's palsy is considered rare but misdiagnosis of Bell's palsy is generally due to ischemic CVA. Most cases spare forehead muscles—advanced age & DM increases this risk[2,3]

No specific testing necessary in most cases of peripheral facial palsy 7th cranial nerve

■ EVALUATION

Determine central from peripheral (central spares forehead muscles on exam)

No testing necessary (labs or imaging) in majority of cases especially new onset[1,4]

Consider imaging (CT/MRI with MRI mode of choice) if symptoms atypical or > 2 months[4]

In bilateral symptoms: CBC, RPR, HIV, BMP for glucose, ANA, Lyme titer, ESR[5]

■ MANAGEMENT

Corneal protection (Lacrilube) & eyelid taping

Corticosteroids (increases the likelihood of restoring function): prednisone 60–80 mg daily for 1 week[6]

Preferable to begin steroids within 3 days of onset

Antivirals (benefits have not been established) combine with steroids[7]

- Acyclovir 800 mg 5 times a day for 7–10 days
- Valaciclovir 1000 mg tid for 7 days

Facial exercise therapy (mime therapy)

In pregnancy:

- Corticosteroids generally safe but has maternal & fetal risks
- Observational studies note corticosteroids are not associated with improvement in pregnancy[8,9]
  - Maternal: DM exacerbation, ulcers, psychosis, fluid retention
  - Fetal: adrenal suppression, low birth weight, defects in the 1st trimester

GENERAL

Self-limited bronchial inflammation is characterized by a cough. May have sputum production. Typical duration is 1–3 weeks

Cannot distinguish between bronchitis & URI before 5 days, but it is not critical to management as both are typically viral[1]

- Acute (1–3 weeks)
- Chronic (COPD associated with a cough at least 3 months in 2 successive years)
- Pneumonia (fever—systemic symptoms)

Sputum color does not demonstrate bacterial infection[2]

Virus most common cause (60% in one study)—bacterial uncommon cause (6% in one study)[3]

EVALUATION

Testing reserved for suspected pneumonia, diagnosis uncertain, or test would change management

CXR unlikely to change management in most instances of an acute cough[4]

CXR indicated only with features suggesting pneumonia (HR > 100, RR > 24, fever, rales, age > 75 yo, ↓O_2 sats)[5]

Procalcitonin (PCT) emerging as an indicator for therapy (more specific bacterial marker than WBC or CRP)[6]

PCT < 0.10 mcg/L=	Strongly discourage antimicrobial
PCT 0.1–0.25 mcg/L=	Discourage antimicrobial
PCT 0.25–0.5 mcg/L=	Encourage antimicrobial
PCT > 0.50 mcg/L=	Strongly encourage antimicrobial

Pertussis testing if suspected for public health[7]

Consider pertussis in apneic infants or severe cough of any duration[8]

Consider other causes of wheezing or a cough:

- ACE inhibitor, GERD, FB aspiration, lung ca, asthma, heart failure, PE, post nasal drip, Strep pharyngitis, influenza

■ MANAGEMENT

Pertussis (a paroxysmal cough) is the only indication for antibiotics to limit spread (particularly pregnant patients)[9,10]

NSAIDs

OTC antihistamine—decongestant

Albuterol MDI only if bronchospasm present[11,12]

Antimicrobial use may be indicated for acute rhino sinusitis (symptoms > 10 days, severe symptoms, fever, facial pain > 3 days or worsening symptoms)[11]

Pertussis treatment:

- Azithromycin 500 mg once, then 250 mg daily for 4 days
- Erythromycin 500 mg QID for 14 days
- Clarithromycin 500 mg BID for 14 days

Consider admission for infants < 6 months with pertussis and respiratory difficulty

Local outbreaks of mycoplasma pneumoniae or chlamydia pneumoniae may consider tetracyclines, macrolides, & fluoroquinolones

☐ GENERAL

CO binds to Hgb greater than O_2 forming carboxyhemoglobin (COHb) inhibiting cellular respiration[1]
  Fetal Hgb has a higher affinity for CO than adults
Even in major CO exposures—COHb levels may be low if several hours have elapsed since exposure[1]
Non-smoker COHb baseline = 3%[2]
Smoker COHb baseline = 10–15%[2]
Severe COPD may result in elevated COHb levels even without tobacco smoke exposure[3]
  Mechanism and clinical significance are unclear[3]
Suspect cyanide (CN) poisoning if there is hemodynamic instability in smoke inhalation patient with serum lactate > 10 mmol/L[4]
CO elimination[5]:
  Room air: 2–7 hours
  100 % O_2: 60–90 minutes
  Hyperbaric oxygen 100% at 3 atm: 23 minutes

■ EVALUATION

Early symptoms resemble flu with the most common being headache[6]
  Malaise, nausea, dizziness—later altered mental status and neurologic symptoms
  Classic "Cherry Red" skin is a late finding generally described post mortem[7]
Neurologic exam/cardiac evaluation:
  Delayed neuropsychiatric syndrome (DNS) cannot be predicted based on COHb level or history[8]
  Myocardial injury is common[9]
Pulse oximetry cannot detect COHb and can be normal even with high levels of CO[10]
Labs:
  COHb level (venous sample can screen, though it is less able to evaluate associated acidosis)[11]
    Typically definitive: > 20%

Suspected: > 10% and associated symptoms (such as headache, vomiting, syncope)
- Levels 10–20% cause headache, nausea, vomiting, dyspnea[12]
- Levels 30–40% cause a severe headache, syncope, tachycardia/arrhythmias[12]
- Levels > 40% cause respiratory failure, seizures, arrest[12]

Blood pH
Serum lactate
CXR
Consider: Chemistries (metabolic abnormalities)
- Troponin (myocardial ischemia)
- Total CK (rhabdomyolysis)
- ECG (if COHb level elevated/confirmed)[9]
- CT head (to assess other causes of neurologic symptoms)
- HCG
- Blood cyanide concentration if concomitant exposure suspected
  - Hydroxycobalamin is the antidote for cyanide poisoning

■ MANAGEMENT

Remove from source: contact a Poison Control Center or toxicologist
High-flow oxygen via face mask
Hyperbaric oxygen[13]:
- COHb level > 25% (> 20% pregnant or evidence of fetal distress)
- Loss of consciousness
- Metabolic acidosis pH < 7.1
- Evidence of end-organ ischemia (chest pain, ECG changes, mental status changes)

No clear discharge guidelines
- Many with mild symptoms can be safely discharged if asymptomatic & COHb < 5%[14]

Psychiatric consultation with self-inflicted cases
Admit if symptoms do not resolve or there is lab evidence of severe poisoning, ECG changes, or other medical/social concerns

Cellulitis

GENERAL

Acute dermal or subcutaneous tissue bacterial infection (includes erysipelas)
- Cellulitis: deeper dermis & subcutaneous layer
- Erysipelas: upper dermis & superficial lymphatics

Typically a clinical diagnosis. Laboratory data may not be needed
- Systemic toxicity must be assessed. Differentiate from necrotizing fasciitis (life-threatening deep fascia) & gas gangrene (both diagnoses suspected clinically & managed surgically)[1]
  - Also consider toxic shock syndrome
- Consider underlying joint, vascular, lymphatic, or inflammatory conditions (septic joints, DVT, osteomyelitis)
- Consider noninfectious such as contact dermatitis, allergy (drug reaction), gout, vasculitis, panniculitis, insect bite, stasis dermatitis, lymphedema, lupus, Kawasaki disease

Etiology: bacterial entry through skin breaches[2]
- Most common organism streptococci (73% frequency)[3,4]
  - Etiology not identified in 27%—but the total response rate is 96% to beta-lactams[4]
- *Staph aureus* (including MRSA) is less common but must be noted[3]
- The most common organism in skin abscesses is *Staph aureus* (75% frequency)[4]

EVALUATION

Typically a clinical diagnosis: erythema, warmth, swelling (erysipelas has raised, clear demarcation and usually is on the face)
- Lab testing typically not required

Cultures of skin or biopsy reserved for atypical cases

Imaging not needed but consider to identify complications (abscess, foreign bodies, gas gangrene)

Blood cultures if extensive involvement, systemic toxicity, comorbidities (DM, lymphedema, immunodeficiency), persistent cellulitis, or atypical exposures (animal bites, contaminants, or water exposures)[4]
- Blood cultures positive in < 10% of cases[5]

Patients with systemic symptoms consider[6]:
- CBC
- Chemistries (creatinine, bicarb)
- CRP
- Blood culture (if sepsis suspected)
- Culture purulent exudates

■ MANAGEMENT

Most approaches target streptococci or modified for MRSA

Mild cellulitis without systemic infection[7,8]
- Pen VK 250–500 mg QID (adults)
- Cephalexin 500 mg BID
- Dicloxacillin 500 mg QID
- Clindamycin 300–450 mg QID
- MRSA:
- Clindamycin 300–450 mg TID
- Trimethoprim/sulfamethoxazole 1 bid *plus* Amoxil 500 mg BID
- Doxycycline 100 mg bid *plus* Amoxicillin 500 mg BID

Cellulitis with systemic signs of infection[6]
- Pen G 2–4 million units IV q 4–6h
- Ceftriaxone 1–2 g IV daily
- Clindamycin 600 mg IV q 8 h
- MRSA:
- Vancomycin 30 mg/kg/d divided BID IV
  - (150 lb = 1 g BID)

Po therapy can be as effective as parenteral therapy[9]

Indications for parenteral instead of po antimicrobials[10–12]:
- Systemic symptoms (fever, tachycardia, hypotension)
- Progression despite 48 hours of po therapy
- Rapid erythema progression
- Inability to tolerate po therapy
- Proximity to indwelling medical device (prosthetic joint, graft)

Consider also in immunocompromised patients
Consider empiric MRSA coverage[12]
(systemic toxicity, lack of response, prior MRSA, exposure to MRSA, proximity indwelling device)

I&D alone generally sufficient for skin abscesses < 2 cm unless[13]:
> 2 cm
Multiple lesions
Immunocompromised or comorbidities
Extensive surrounding cellulitis
Systemic symptoms
Presence of indwelling device (prosthetic join, pacemaker, graft)
Insufficient response to I&D
High risk of transmission (prison inmates, athletes, military)

19 COPD

GENERAL

Airflow obstruction with chronic inflammatory response resulting in lung tissue destruction[1]

Typically > 40 yo of age patients with smoking as a common risk factor

Sub-types = emphysema, chronic bronchitis, chronic obstructive asthma, emphysema

There are technical interrelationships between subtypes

Alpha-1 antitrypsin deficiency is a hereditary cause (consider testing if symptoms persist over time)[2]

Especially young adults or nonsmokers, though not an ER issue

Has risk factors for respiratory irritant exposure (tobacco use)[3]

Most common symptom triad of dyspnea, chronic cough, and sputum production[3]

Common early symptom is exertional dyspnea[4]

Early disease may have a normal exam. Prolonged expiratory phase or wheezing on forced exhalation

As severity increases hyperinflation occurs with decreased breath sounds, wheezes, or crackles at lung base[5]

EVALUATION

No single test diagnostic but can exclude other causes of dyspnea

Pulmonary function tests (PFTs—spirometry) are the most objective standard for confirmation of the diagnosis[3,6]

Severity	Postbronchodilator FEV_1
GOLD 1 (mild)	> 80% predicted
GOLD 2 (moderate)	50% to < 80% predicted
GOLD 3 (severe)	> 30% to < 50% predicted
GOLD 4 (very severe)	< 30% predicted

CBC
Chemistries—elevated serum bicarb may aid in identifying chronic hypercapnia
BNP (suspected heart failure)
Cardiac enzymes (suspected ischemia)
CXR
Echocardiogram & EKG if cor pulmonale suspected
Pulse oximetry
 Supplemental O_2 not necessary if saturation > 90%
 Does not provide data on alveolar ventilation or hypercapnia so may be inaccurate in COPD setting[7]
Arterial blood gas (ABG) in certain situations (poor spirometry, mental status change, low saturation)

■ MANAGEMENT

No single medication alters the decline of long-term lung function. Goal of therapy is to reduce symptoms & complications
Bronchodilators (albuterol) including ipratropium
Corticosteroids
Macrolides (azithromycin)
 Antibiotic may have anti-inflammatory effect[8,9]
 IV antibiotics may reduce treatment failure in severe patients[10]
Theophylline (less used—toxicity can occur)
Mucolytics (little evidence of effectiveness)
Oxygen
No benefit demonstrated from Heliox[11]
Magnesium sulfate 1-2 g IV[12]
Nebulized saline[13]
Admit:
 Severe symptoms
  Resting dyspnea, elevated respiratory rate, mental status change, low saturations, serious comorbidities, poor social support[3]

☐ GENERAL

Corneal epithelium defect typically due to trauma[1]
    Pain, photophobia, and/or foreign body sensation
Etiologies include: trauma, contact lens, chemical/radiation burns, FBs, airbags[1]
    Most heal in 24–72 hours

■ EVALUATION

Assess for penetrating trauma & infectious etiology
    CT orbit if an open globe is suspected, intraocular FB, or intraorbital hemorrhage[2]
Globe rupture findings: marked decrease visual acuity—eccentric pupil—low intraocular pressure (IOP)—vitreous extrusion
    Tenting defect at globe injury site—prolapsed ocular structures—Seidel's sign (teardrop stream pattern)—significant change in the globe contour
Exam (typically aided by topical anesthetic)[1]
    Visual acuity
    Invert eyelids (for FB)
        Sweep surface with moistened cotton swab
    Pupil reaction to light & fundus exam
    Check for hyphema
    Location of hyperemia
    Corneal appearance (hazy, inflammation, injection, FBs)
    Consider measurement of the intraocular pressure **if you do not suspect an open globe**
        Increased IOP occurs often after hyphema[3]
    Fluorescein stain exam with Wood's Lamp or Cobalt Blue Filter (perform last)
Fluorescein exam confirms diagnosis
    Watch for Seidel's sign (fluorescein streaming caused by aqueous humor leakage indicating penetrating trauma)
    Branching pattern may indicate herpes zoster ophthalmicus or healing abrasion[1]
Slit-lamp patterns[1]:
    Contact lens—punctate abrasions
    Traumatic—linear, mechanical shape

Penetrating trauma—Seidel sign, hyphema
Herpetic—branching (dendritic) appearance
Flash burn—numerous punctate lesions over entire corneal surface
Lid FB—multiple vertical lines

MANAGEMENT

Globe penetration requires emergent ophthalmology consultation[1,4]
Hyphema requires prompt ophthalmology consultation as the majority of cases have injury to other ocular structures[4]
Corneal abrasions need prompt ophthalmology consultation if[1,4]:
- Ulceration is suggested by white spot, infiltrate, or opacity
- Pus (hypopyon) in anterior chamber
- FB that cannot be removed

Referral to ophthalmologist[1,4]:
- Symptoms persist > 48–72 hours
- Large abrasions (> 50% corneal surface area)
- Rust ring
- Chemical burn (needs copious irrigation)
- Defect over visual axis

Artificial tears[1]
Despite recent studies—topical anesthetics beyond exam period remain controversial[5,6]
Opioids in severe cases
Corticosteroids contraindicated[1]
Topical cycloplegics only considered in cases of traumatic iritis[1]
Topical antimicrobials often prescribed with limited evidence of efficacy[1]
- Contact lens patients—ciprofloxacin or ofloxacin for antipseudomonal activity[1]
- Ointment may be more lubricating than gtts[1]
  - Erythromycin ointment 0.5%
  - Sulfacetamide ointment 10%
  - Bacitracin/polymyxin B ointment
  - Bacitracin ointment

Little evidence that patching eye has utility.[1,7]

Ketorolac 0.5% 1 gtt QID may reduce pain[1,8]
  There is some controversy regarding complications
  Do not use in contact lens users or bleeding disorders
Consider Td prophylaxis
Follow-up may not be needed if abrasion is small (< 4 mm), normal vision, uncomplicated course, & symptoms resolving[1]
Do not wear contact lens until the cornea is completely healed
Follow-up with ophthalmology in 24 hours if the injury is due to contacts, fingernail, organic material, or large abrasion[1]
  To assess for complications, corneal ulcer, infection, or erosion

LARYNGOTRACHEOBRONCHITIS

☐ GENERAL

Classically noted by barking cough
  Parainfluenza virus the most common etiology[1]
DDx: croup, uvulitis, bacterial tracheitis, peritonsilar or retropharyngeal infection, angioedema, foreign bodies, diptheria, epiglottitis, allergic reaction, congential anomaly[2]

■ EVALUATION

Assess severity
  Westley Croup Score[3]
    LOC: normal (including sleep) = 0; disoriented = 5
    Cyanosis: none = 0; with agitation = 4; at rest = 5
    Stridor: none = 0; with agitation = 1; at rest = 2
    Air entry: normal = 0; decreased = 1; markedly decreased = 2
    Retractions: none = 0; mild = 1; moderate = 2; severe = 3
Soft tissue neck/CXR if unclear Dx[4]
  Croup: steeple sign with subglottic STS
  Epiglottitis: thumbprint sign with epiglottitis STS
Labs generally not indicated[5]
  CBC (viral pattern typically)[6]

■ MANAGEMENT

Westley Croup Score
Mild: < or = 2 (bark cough, hoarse cry, no rest stridor, no retractions)
  Mild Tx: **humidity, fever control, po fluids** (consider dexamethasone 0.6 mg/kg [max 10 mg] single dose by least invasive method). Outpatient Tx
Mod: 3–7 (stridor at rest, may have mild retractions, no agitation)
  Mod Tx: **Same as below**—outpatient Tx unless Sx persist
Severe: ≥ 8 (Sig. rest stridor, severe retractions, anxious)
  Mod-Severe Tx: **pulse ox, consider IVFs, aerosolized racemic epi** (can be repeated q 15 min), **dexamethasone (0.6 mg/kg, max 10 mg) by the least invasive method**

Observe mod-severe 3–4 hours

If patient remains comfortable may be discharged home if meet following criteria: No stridor at rest, NL pulse ox, good air exchange, NL color, NL level of consciousness, demonstrates the ability to tolerate po fluid, caregivers understand return indications[7]

INDICATIONS FOR ADMISSION

Need for supplemental O_2, mod retractions & tachypnea, toxicity, poor po intake, age particularly under 6 months, 24-hour ER return, family compliance concerns[7,8]

Heliox[9]

Evidence of short-term benefit

Prognosis: symptoms usually resolve in 3 days to 1 week. Up to 15% require hospitalization & among those 1% require intubation[10,11]

☐ GENERAL

Maintain cervical immobilization until an unstable spinal injury is excluded.

Removing the patient from the backboard and placing the patient on a stretcher while maintaining c-spine immobilization prevents complications[1]

- No evidence that backboards improve outcomes & they are associated with complications
- Backboards also cause neck flexion in children < 8 yo who have larger heads

Spinal injury is rare in penetrating trauma & in the absence of evidence suggesting neurologic injury[2]

■ EVALUATION

Canadian C-Spine Rule[3]

Determines the need for imaging in blunt trauma to head or neck

Use only on alert, stable patients (Glasgow Coma score 15)

Patients < 16 yo excluded

Perform x-ray if any of the following high-risk characteristics are present (Condition 1):

- *Age over 65 yo (consider CT > 65 yo)[4]*
- *Dangerous mechanism of injury (fall > 3 ft or 5 stairs, axial load, high-speed MVC (> 62 mph/100 kmh, rollover, ejection, ATV accident, bike collision)*
- *Paresthesias to extremities*

If above high risk not found in Condition 1—assess for low-risk ROM assessment (Condition 2):

- *Rear end collisions (simple: excluding high impact by larger vehicle)*
- *Ambulatory at any time since the injury*
- *Able to sit in ER*
- *Delayed onset of neck pain*
- *No midline cervical spine tenderness*

X-ray those who do not meet Condition 2 risk factors

Perform ROM assessment for those who do meet Condition 2 risk factors

No x-ray needed if able to rotate 45° in each direction left & right regardless of pain (Condition 3)

X-ray if unable to assess

Nexus **Low-Risk Criteria**[5,6]

Does not apply to age > 60 yo

May be less sensitive in patients age < 8 yo[7]

X-ray not needed if all 5 criteria are present:

1. *No posterior midline cervical tenderness*
2. *Normal alertness level in ER*
   Brief LOC at time of MVC does not preclude applying rule, as long as all other criteria met[8]
3. *No evidence of intoxication*
4. *No abnormal neurologic findings*
5. *No painful distracting injuries present*
   Distracting = long bone fractures, visceral injury requiring surgical consultation, large lacerations, crush injury, large burns, or any injury as to impair the ability to appreciate other injuries

Consider x-ray as first-line evaluation for low risk[5]

Consider CT as first-line evaluation for high suspicion or multiple trauma[9]

Consider MRI for suspected soft tissue or cord injury & neurologic abnormalities despite normal CT[5]

MANAGEMENT

Neurosurgery consult

Stabilize spine & maintain the airway

Treat shock as a result of hemorrhage or neurogenic in origin

In neurogenic shock steroid administration is the only suggested treatment improving outcome; however, the evidence is still limited and controversial[10]

For Alert and Stable Trauma Patients

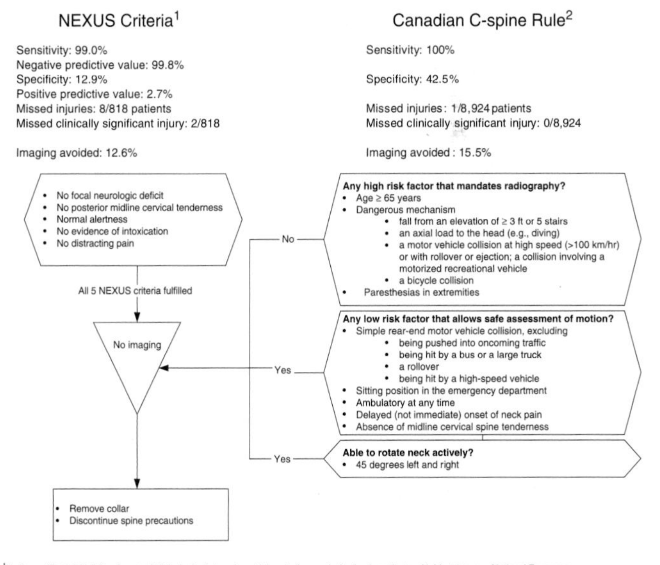

[1]Hoffman JR et al. Validity of a set of clinical criteria to rule out injury to the cervical spine in patients with blunt trauma. National Emergency X-Radiography Utilization Study Group. N Engl J Med 2000;343.

[2]Stiell IG et al. The Canadian C-spine rule for radiography in alert and stable trauma patients. JAMA 2001;286:1841.

☐ GENERAL

Establish airway, breathing, circulation (ABC)[1]
  Intubate if necessary
  Oxygen should not be given to non-hypoxic patients (saturation > 94%)[1]
Determine the time of onset to assess candidates for thrombolytic or thrombectomy[1]
  If unclear—onset is defined as last time awake & symptom free[1]
ABCD rule for CVA prediction within 7 days of TIA[2]

Age	> 60 y	1 point
BP	Sys > 140 mm Hg and/or Dias > 90 mm Hg	1 point
Clinical	Unilateral weakness	2 points
	Speech impaired but no weakness	1 point
	None	0 points
Duration	> 60 mins	2 points
	10–59 mins	1 point
	< 10 mins	0 points

Score	0–3 points	Minimal CVA risk within 7 days
	4 points	1.1–9.1% 7-day risk
	5 points	12–16% 7-day risk
	6 points	24–36% 7-day risk

■ EVALUATION

Stat head CT (differentiate ischemic from hemorrhagic)[1,3]
Stat finger stick glucose[1,3]
Stat oxygen saturation[1,3]
Stat neuro logic consult
Document NIH Stroke Score

Establish candidacy for thrombolytic or thrombectomy therapy[1,3]

Therapeutic window = 4.5 hours from onset of symptoms

Inclusion criteria

Ischemic CVA with measurable neuro deficit

Onset < 4.5 hours

If DM or previous CVA: 3 hours

> 18 yo

Exclusion criteria

Previous IC bleed

CVA or head trauma within 3 months

IC neoplasm, AV malformation, or aneurysm

Recent IC or spinal surgery

Arterial puncture past 7 days

Subarachnoid hemorrhage symptoms

Glucose < 50 mg/dL

BP > 185 systolic or > 110 diastolic

Active internal bleeding or bleeding diathesis

- Platelet count < 100,000/mm^3

Current anticoagulation use with INR > 1.7 or thrombin inhibitor with evidence of anticoagulation effect on INR or assays

Heparin use past 48 hours

Head CT shows evidence of hemorrhage or extensive regions of obvious hypodensity consistent with irreversible injury

Relative exclusion criteria

Minor or isolated neurologic symptoms

Rapidly improving symptoms

Major surgery previous 14 days

GI bleed/hematuria past 21 days

MI past 3 months

Seizure at stroke onset

Pregnancy

If time 3–4.5 hours relative exclusion

Age > 80 yo

Po anticoagulation use regardless of INR

Severe stroke (NIHSS score > 25)

Combo of both previous CVA & DM

Labs[1,3]	Below labs in certain cases
CBC	Toxicology
Chemistry panel	ETOH
PT/INR, PPT	HCG
Cardiac enzymes	ABG
ECG	CXR
U/A	LP (if SAH suspected & CT head neg)

■ MANAGEMENT

Stabilize Airway, Breathing, Circulation
Head of bed (HOB) 30°[4]
BP management research is limited to first 24 hours of CVA
- Ischemic: goal to be eligible for thrombolytics: < 185/110 & maintained there for 24 hrs after treatment[1]
  - Labetalol 10–20 mg IV over 2 minutes (may repeat once) or
  - Nicardipine 5 mg/h IV titrate up by 2.5 mg/h every 5–15 minutes when necessary (PRN) (max 15 mg/h)
- Ischemic: non-thrombolytic candidate's BP treated if extreme (> 220/120) or has active CAD, renal failure, or preeclampsia[1]
- Hemorrhagic: balance risk (reducing perfusion) with the benefit (reducing further bleeding) —in general, lower systolic BP to around 130–140
  - Labetalol & nicardipine first line if needed as titratable agents[1]
- Consider hypertensive encephalopathy (mimics CVA) in which decrease BP is the treatment

Fluid management: normal saline. Avoid hypotonic ½ NS as it may exacerbate edema[5]
IC bleeds: reverse any anticoagulation[6]
- Vitamin K 1–10 mg PO or slow IV
- Fresh frozen plasma (FFP) but may require up to 8 units
- Prothrombin-complex concentrate

Admission to Stroke Center may decrease mortality & may have further interventions such as thrombectomy treatment.[7]

NIH Stroke Scale

Instructions	Scale Defenition	Score
1a. Level of consciousness: The investigator must choose aresponse, even if a full evaluation is prevented by such obstacles as an endotracheal tube, language barrier, orotracheal trauma/bandages. A "3" is scored only if the patient makes no movement (other than reflexive posturing) in response to noxious stimulation.	0 = Alert; keenly responsive 1 = Not alert, but arousable by minor stimulation to obey, answer, or respond 2 = Not alert, requires repeated stimulation to attend, or is obtunded and requires strong or painful stimulation to make movements (not stereotyped) 3= Responds only with reflect motor or autonomic effects or totally unresponsive, flaccid, areflexic	______
1b. LOC Questions: The patient is asked the month and his/her age. The answer must be correct - there is no partial credit for being close. Aphasic and stuporous patients who do not comprehend the questions will score "2." Patients unable to speak because of endotracheal intubation, orotracheal trauma, severe dysarthia from any cause, language barrier or any other problem not secondary to aphasia are given a "1." **It is important that only the initial answer be graded and that the examiner not "help" the patient with verbal or non-verbal cues.**	0 = Answers both questions correctly 1 = Answers one question correctly 2 = Answers neither question correctly	______
1c. LOC Commands: The patient is asked to open and close the eyes and then to grip and release the non-paretic hand. Substitute another one-step command if the hands cannot be used. Credit is given if an unequivocal attempt is made but not completed due to weakness. **If the patient does not respond to commands, the task should be demonstrated to them (pantomime)** and score the result (i.e., follows none, one or two commands). Patients with trauma, amputation, or other physical impediments should be given suitable one-step commands. Only the first attempt is scored.	0 = Performs both tasks correctly 1 = Performs one task correctly 2 = Performs neither task correctly	______

(Continued)

NIH Stroke Scale - Continued

Instructions	Scale Defenition	Score
2. Best Gaze: Only horizontal eye movements will be tested. Voluntary or reflexive (oculocephalic) eye movements will be scored but calorie testing is not done. If the patient has a conjugate deviation of the eyes that can be overcome by voluntary or reflexive activity, the score will be "1." If a patient has an isolated peripheral nerve paresis (CN, III, IV or VI) score a "1." Gaze is testable in all aphasic patients. Patients with ocular trauma, bandages, pre-existing blindness or other disorder of visual acuity or fields should be tested with reflexive movements and a choice made by the investigator. Establishing eye contact and then moving about the patient from side to side will occasionally clarify the presence of a partial gaze palsy.	0 = Normal 1 = Partial gaze palsy. This score is given when gaze is abnormal in one or both eyes, but where forced deviation or total gaze paresis are not present 2 = Forced deviation, or total gaze paresis not overcome by the oculocephalic maneuver	______
3. Visual: Visual fields (upper and lower quadrants) are tested by confrontation, using finger counting or visual threat as appropriate. Patient must be encouraged, but if they look at the side of the moving fingers appropriately, this can be scored as normal. If there is unilateral blindness or enucleation, visual fields in the remaining eye are scored. Score 1 only if a clear-cut asymmetry, including quadrant anopia is found. If patient is blind from any cause, score "3." Double simultaneous stimulation is performed at this point. **If there is extinction, patient receives a "1" and the results are used to answer question #11.**	0 = No visual loss 1 = Partial hemianopia 2 = Complete hemianopia 3 = Bilateral hemianopia (blind, including cortical blindness)	______
4. Facial Palsy: Ask, or use pantomime to encourage the patient to show teeth or raise eyebrows and close eyes. Score symmetry of grimace in response to noxious stimuli in the poorly responsive or non-comprehending patient. If facial trauma/bandages, orotracheal tube, tape or other physical barrier obscures the face, these should be removed to the extent possible.	0 = Normal symmetrical movement 1 = Minor paralysis (flattened nasolabial fold, asymmetry on smiling) 2 = Partial paralysis (total or near total paralysis of lower face) 3 = Complete paralysis of one or both sides (absence of facial movement in the upper and lower face)	______

(Continued)

NIH Stroke Scale - Continued

<table>
<tr><th>Instructions</th><th>Scale Defenition</th><th>Score</th></tr>
<tr><td rowspan="2">5 & 6. Motor Arm and Leg: The limb is placed in the appropriate position: extend the arms (palms down) 90 degrees (if sitting) or 45 degrees (if supine) and the leg 30 degrees (always tested supine). Drift is scored if the arm falls before 10 seconds or the leg before 5 seconds. The aphasic patient is encouraged using urgency in the voice and pantomime but not noxious stimulation. Each limb is tested in turn, beginning with the non-paretic arm. Only in the case of amputation or joint fusion at the shoulder or hip may the score be "9" and the examiner must clearly write the explanation for scoring as a "9".</td><td>0 = No drift, limb holds 90 (or 45) degrees for full 10 seconds
1 = Drift, Limb holds 90 (or 45) degrees, but drifts down before full 10 seconds; does not hit bed or other support
2 = Some effort against gravity, limb cannot get to or maintain (if cued) 90 (or 45) degrees, drifts down to bed, but has some effort against gravity
3 = No effort against gravity, limb falls
4 = No movement
9 = Amputation, joint fusion; explain: ____ ________
5a. Left Arm.......................................
5b. Right Arm....................................</td><td>

____
________</td></tr>
<tr><td>0 = No drift, leg holds 30 degrees position for full 5seconds.
1 = Drift, leg falls by the end of the 5 second period but does not hit bed.
2 = Some effort against gravity; leg falls to bed by 5 seconds, but has some effort against gravity.
3 = No effort against gravity, leg falls to bed immediately.
4 = No movement
9 = Amputation, joint fusion explain:____ ________
6a. Left Leg.......................................
6b. Right Leg....................................</td><td>

____
________</td></tr>
</table>

(Continued)

NIH Stroke Scale - Continued

Instructions	Scale Defenition	Score
7. Limb Ataxia: This item is aimed at finding evidence of a unilateral cerebellar lesion. Test with eyes open. In case of visual defect, insure testing is done in intact visual field. The finger-nose-finger and heel-shin tests are performed on both sides, and ataxia is scored only if present out of proportion to weakness. Ataxia is absent in the patient who cannot understand or is paralyzed. Only in the case of amputation or joint fusion may the item be scored "9", and the examiner must clearly write the explanation for not scoring. In case of blindness test by touching nose from extended arm position.	0 = Absent 1 = Present in one limb 2 = Present in two limbs	______
8. Sensory: Sensation or grimace to pin prick when tested, or withdrawal from noxious stimulus in the obtunded or aphasic patient. Only sensory loss attributed to stroke is scored as abnormal and the examiner should test as many body areas [arms (not hands), legs, trunk, face] as needed to accurately check for hemisensory loss. A score of 2, "severe or total," should only be given when a severe or total loss of sensation can be clearly demonstrated. Stuporous and aphasic patients will therefore probably score 1 or 0. The patient with brain stem stroke who has bilateral loss of sensation is scored 2. If the patient does not respond and is quadriplegic score 2. Patients in coma (item 1a=3) are arbitrarily given a 2 on this item.	0 = Normal; no sensory loss 1 = Mild to moderate sensory loss; patient feels pinprick is less sharp or is dull on the affected s side; or there is a loss of superficial pain with pinprick but patient is aware he/she is being touched 2 = Severe to total sensory loss; patient is not aware of being touched in the face, arm and leg	______

(Continued)

NIH Stroke Scale - Continued

Instructions	Scale Defenition	Score
9. Best Language: A great deal of information about comprehension will be obtained during the preceding sections of the examination. The patient is asked to describe what is happening in the attached picture, to name the items on the attached naming sheet, and to read from the attached list of sentences. Comprehension is judged from responses here as well as to all of the commands in the preceding general neurological exam. If visual loss interferes with the tests, ask the patient to identify objects placed in the hand, repeat, and produce speech. The intubated patient should be asked to write. The patient in coma (question 1a=3) will arbitrarily score 3 on this item. The examiner must choose a score in the patient with stupor or limited cooperation but a score of 3 should be used only if the patient is mute and follows no one step commands.	0 = No aphasia, normal 1 = Mild to moderate aphasia; some obvious loss of fluency or facility of comprehension, without significant limitation on ideas expressed or form of expression. Reduction of speech and/or comprehension, however, makes conversation about provided material difficult or impossible. For example, in conversation about provided materials examiner can identify picture or naming card from patient's response. 2 = Severe aphasia; all communication is through fragmentary expression; great need for inference, questioning and guessing by the listener. Range of information that can be exchanged is limited; listener carries burden of communication. Examiner cannot identify materials provided from patient response. 3 = Mute, global aphasia; no usable speech or auditory comprehension	______
10. Dysarthria: If patient is thought to be normal an adequate sample of speech must be obtained by asking patient to read or repeat words from the attached list. If the patient has severe aphasia, the clarity of articulation of spontaneous speech can be rated. Only if the patient is intubated or has other physical barrier to producing speech, may the item be scored "9", and the examiner must clearly write an explanation for not scoring. Do not tell the patient why he/she is being tested.	0 = Normal 1 = Mild to moderate; patient slurs at least some words and, at worst, can be understood with some difficulty 2 = Severe; patient's speech is so slurred as to be unintelligible in the absence of or out of proportion to any dysphasia, or is mute/anarthric 9 = Intubated or other physical barrier, explain	______

(Continued)

NIH Stroke Scale - Continued

Instructions	Scale Defenition	Score
11. Extinction and Inattention (formerly Neglect): Sufficient information to identify neglect may be obtained during the prior testing. If the patient has a severe visual loss preventing visual double simultaneous stimulation, and the cutaneous stimuli are normal, the score is normal. If the patient has aphasia but does appear to attend to both sides, the score is normal. The presence of visual spatial neglector anosognosia may also be taken as evidence of abnormality. Since the abnormality is scored only if present, the item is never untestable.	0 = No abnormality 1 = Visual, tactile, auditory, spatial, or personal inattention or extinction to bilateral simultaneous stimulation in one of the sensory modalities 2 = Profound hemi-inattention or hemi-inattention to more than one modality. Does not recognize own hand or orients to only one side of space.	______
	Total NIHSS Score:	

Time of NIHSS Assessment:______________
Date of NIHSS Assessment:______________
Physician/NIHSS Certified Individual Signature: ______________________________

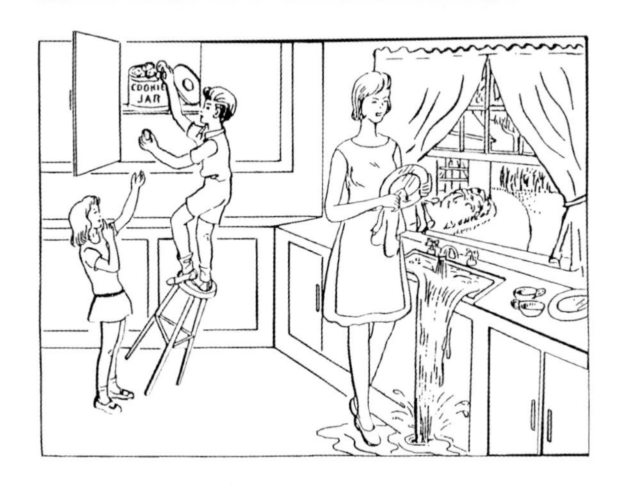

Down to earth.

I got home from work.

Near the table in the dining room.

They heard him speak on the radio last night.

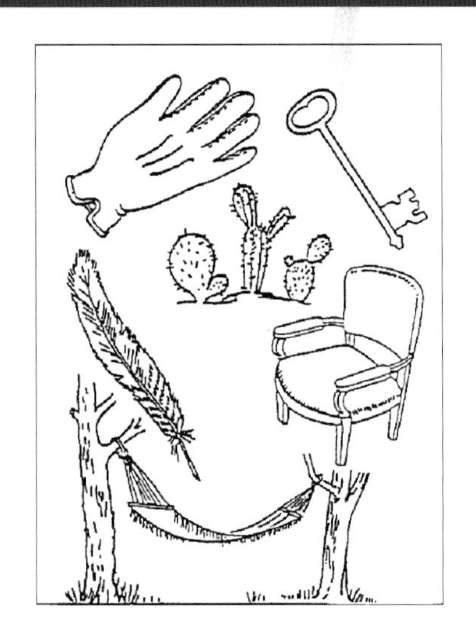

MAMA

TIP – TOP

FIFTY – FIFTY

THANKS

HUCKLEBERRY

BASEBALL PLAYER

☐ GENERAL

Idiopathic process denoted by recurrent vomiting with intervening periods of normal health[1]
- Vomiting 3 or more episodes[2,3]
- Normal health between episodes[2,3]
- Stereotypical episodes of onset, timing, symptoms, & duration[2,3]
- No organic cause identified[3]

Trigger mechanisms can be identified in 68–80% of episodes[4]

Chronic cannabis use is a leading trigger[5]
- Cannabis hyperemesis syndrome may be a separate diagnosis

There may be an association between migraines, abdominal migraines, & CVS[6]

■ EVALUATION

An observation period & exclusion of other serious causes (ie, brain tumors, volvulus) is needed[7]
- Patients with cannabis trigger will self-medicate with cannabis to control emesis
- If patient avoids cannabis for 1–2 weeks & still experiences emesis—continue CVS evaluation[8]
- Ask about frequent bathing behavior—it is often present in cannabis abuse (ie, hot showers)

Rome IV criteria[9]:
- Typical episodes of acute vomiting < 1-week duration
- Three or more episodes in the past year & 2 in past 6 months at least a week apart
- No vomiting between episodes

Family or personal history of migraine is supportive criteria

No specific lab testing—avoid broad testing but target the evaluation if any of the following markers are present[10]:
- Abdominal signs (bilious vomiting, tenderness, unilateral pain)
- Triggers (fasting, high-protein meal, signs of illness)
- Abnormal neurologic findings (altered mental status, severe headaches)
- Worsening or changing pattern of episodes

Chemistries for electrolytes, glucose, BUN, creatinine[10]

Abdominal films for malrotation of bowe[10]

Lactic acid may be increased during an acute episode[10]
U/A (ketosis may be present)
Lipase[10]
CT abdomen/pelvis may be warranted if alarming signs are present[10]
Consider brain MRI if neurologic signs are present
Ammonia if illness, fasting, or a high-protein meal is the trigger
If hyponatremia or hypoglycemia present—consider an Addison's disease evaluation[10]

■ MANAGEMENT

Admission if continuous IVF, antiemetics, or occasional analgesics required
- Refer children to a specialist such as a pediatric GI or neurologist as needed

No specific effective treatment has been identified[11]
- Antimigraine medication trial has been suggested
- Sumatriptan—propranolol—tricyclic antidepressants (po dosing)[12]
  - Amitriptyline > age 5 yo start 0.5 mg/kg per day qhs[13]
    - May require 1 mg/kg qhs & 1–2 months to effect[13]
    - Median adult dose 50 mg daily[14]
  - Doxepin has also been used

Over-the-counter coenzyme Q10 & L-carnitine dietary supplements[15]
Ondansetron 0.15 mg/kg IV q 4 h up to 3 doses[16]
- (do not exceed 16 mg single dose IV or 8 mg > age 75 yo due to the risk of QT prolongation)[16]
- High-dose ondansetron (0.3 mg/kg dose max 20 mg) has been described (see FDA warnings)

Sedation by adding lorazepam or diphenhydramine may be needed
Consider Haloperidol
Dextrose 10% with 0.45% NS IV has been added with anecdotal success

□ GENERAL

Most infections have mixed organisms[1]

Differentiate from more serious infections (peritonsillar abscess, parotid gland infections, Ludwig's angina, or other face or deep neck infections) that could spread intracranially or cause airway compromise[2]

■ EVALUATION

Consider non-dental source (such as sinusitis, TMJ, neuralgia, OM, parotitis, ulcers, pericoronitis, sialolithiasis, arteritis)

CT imaging is the technique of choice if there is concern for deep face or neck involvement[3]

- Lateral x-ray neck may reveal any tracheal compression/retropharyngeal abnormality

Lab testing is generally not indicated[1]

- CBC/CRP may suggest extension

■ MANAGEMENT

Refer to dentist

Consider avoiding monotherapy for serious infections as failures occur[4]

IV therapy

- Ampicillin-sulbactam 3 g IV or
- Pen G 2–4 million units plus metronidazole 500 mg IV or
- Clindamycin 600 mg IV

Po therapy

- Pen VK 500 mg QID
- Amoxicillin/clavulanic acid 875 mg BID
- Clindamycin 450 mg TID

Pain management

- Combination formulations of acetaminophen & ibuprofen have demonstrated benefit[5]
- Consider po topical formulations: Maalox : Viscous Lidocaine : Diphenhydramine
- NSAIDs recommended before opioids[6]

Antimicrobial therapy recommendations & utility variable[7]

25 Dental Abscess

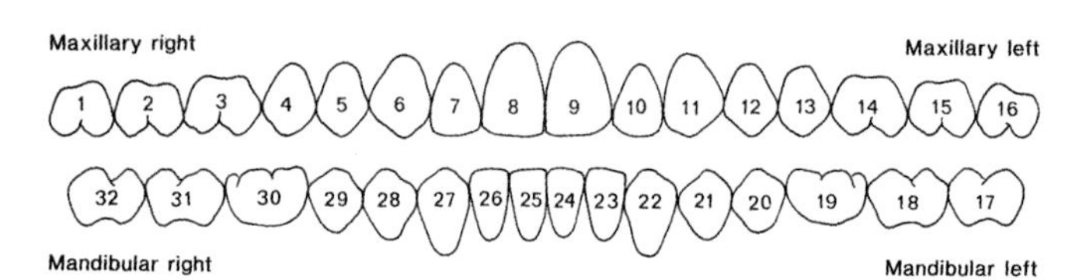

Maxillary right Maxillary left

A B C D E F G H I J

T S R Q P O N M L K

Mandibular right Mandibular left

☐ GENERAL

Earliest hyperglycemia symptoms: polyruria, polydipsia, weight loss
Early ketoacidosis symptoms: abdominal pain, nausea, vomiting, hyperventilation
DKA (and hyperosmolar hyperglycemic state–HHS) is characterized by[1]:
  Serum glucose > 250 mg/dL (HHS > 600)
  Serum bicarb < 18 mEq/L (HHS > 18)
  Anion gap > 10 (HHS variable)
  Blood pH < 7.30 (HHS > 7.30)
  Elevated serum/urine ketones (HHS small)
  Dehydration
Differentiate from hyperosmolar hyperglycemic crisis
  Glucose generally higher in HHS (> 600)—pH > 7.3—bicarb > 18—small ketones—osmolality > 320 mOsm/kg
DKA: triad of hyperglycemia, anion gap metabolic acidosis, ketonemia[2]
HHS: profound hyperglycemia, little ketoacid, increased serum osmolality, frequent neurologic abnormalities[2]
Symptoms of DKA: Kussmaul deep respirations, fruity breath odor, dehydration, mental status change

■ EVALUATION

Labs:
  Chemistry—include magnesium & phosphate[3]
  CBC, U/A, and ECG
  ABG if bicarb reduced or hypoxia suspected
  HbA1c useful to differentiate control history of DM
  Serum beta-hydroxybutyrate[4]
  Blood cultures if sepsis suspected
  CXR if pneumonia suspected

■ MANAGEMENT

Monitor glucose hourly & electrolytes, venous pH every 2–4 hours until stable
Treat any underlying causes: UTI, MI, infections

IVF[5]:

Severe hypovolemia: IV NS 0.9% (adult ~ 1 L/h) for first several hours

Mild hypovolemia: assess corrected serum sodium for IVF management

(For every glucose 100 mg/dL > 100, add 2 mEq to sodium value)

Mild hypovolemia without hyponatremia = 250–500 mL/h 0.45% NS

Mild hypovolemia with hyponatremia = 250–500 mL/h 0.9% NS

When glucose achieves 200, switch IVF to 5% dextrose with 0.45% at 150–250 mL/h

Insulin[5]:

Bolus 0.1 units/kg IV then infuse 0.1 units/kg/h (150 lbs = 8–10 units bolus & 7 units/h infusion)

OR

0.14 units/kg/h without bolus[6]

SC insulin just as effective as IV in DKA (initial 0.3 units/kg followed by 0.1 units/kg qh until glucose < 250) for stable patients & only with adequate nursing staffing to monitor hourly[7,8]

K^+[5]:

Ensure urine output > 50 mL/h

K^+ < 3.3 mEq/L = use 20–40 KCL mEq/h added to IV & **replace K^+ prior to starting insulin (insulin would worsen hypokalemia)**[9]

K^+ 3.3–5.2 mEq/L = use 20–30 KCL mEq/h/L of IVF

K^+> 5.3 = do not give K^+ but monitor every 2 hours

Consider magnesium sulfate supplementation (8–12 g IV first 24 hours)[10]

Bicarb: 100 mmol (100 mEq) $NaHCO_3$ in 400 mL H_2O over 2 hours only if pH < 6.9 infuse over 2 hours[5]

Cerebral edema is a complication mostly in < 20-yo patients[11,12]

Symptoms can occur 12–24 hours after initiation of treatment due to osmolar shifts

1–2 L NS generally safe in adults

Monitor children closely—they do not receive a bolus of insulin (only an insulin drip) and in general fluid requirements are less

Mannitol (0.25–1 g/kg) may be helpful in cerebral edema cases[11]

Admit severe cases to the ICU

GENERAL

Acute, constant abd pain typically in the LLQ[1]
- N/V, low-grade fever, po intake intolerance, & peritonitis symptoms may be present[1]

< 2% of diverticulitis perforate[2]
- Perforation increases mortality rate to approximately 20%[2]

EVALUATION

CBC (WBC may be normal in 45% of cases)[3]
Chemistries
U/A
HCG in females
Suspected perforation: liver functions—alkaline phosphatase—direct bilirubin—lipase
Hemoccult stool[4]
Abdominal CT (po & IV contrast) has 94% sensitivity & 99% specificity[5]
- However, most radiologists are fine with no PO contrast and it can be picked up on a renal protocol CT as well

CT is the most common test to confirm the diagnosis, though it may not be necessary in mild cases[4]

MANAGEMENT

Outpatient management is a safe option in uncomplicated cases[6]
Inpatient management[7]
- Complicated cases: fistula, obstruction, abscess, perforation
- Other cases including sepsis, immunosuppression (such as uncontrolled DM, HIV), fever > 102.5°F, advanced age, significant leukocytosis, significant abdominal pain or comorbidities, intolerance to po intake, unreliability, failed outpatient management

Outpatient treatment with antibiotics—reevaluate in 2–3 days—admit if not improving[8]
- Antimicrobial options Tx 10-14 days (consult local antibiogram):
  - Trimethoprim/sulfamethoxazole BID plus metronidazole 500 mg TID or QID
  - Ciprofloxacin 500 mg BID plus metronidazole 500 mg TID or QID

Amoxicillin/clavulanic acid 875 mg BID
Levofloxacin 750 mg daily plus metronidazole 500 mg TID or QID
Piperacillin–azobactam 3.375 g IV q 6 h
Ticarcillin–clavulanate 3.1 g IV q 6 h
Imipenen–cilastatin 500 mg q 6 h

Colonoscopy after resolution[9]

GENERAL

Most common in children—can occur at any age[1]
  Infants (age < 1 yo) & advanced age (age > 85 yo) are most vulnerable[2]
Haemophilus influenza type b (Hib) most common etiology in children[3]
  Routine immunization has decreased the incidence significantly, although it still occurs[3]
Wide range of causes in adults—bacteria, virus, and mixed—many have negative cultures[4]
  Strep is noted as a key etiology[5]
Medical emergency: respiratory distress—stridor—anxiety—tripod posture—will not lie down—drooling—"hot potato" voice
  Unimmunized, underimmunized, or immunocompromised are major risk factors

EVALUATION

Onset may be abrupt—defer direct visualization or painful procedures until after airway assessment[6]
  Posture may indicate partial obstruction—high fever—dyspnea—muffled voice—sore throat[2]
  Secure airway if respiratory distress is present before other diagnostics[2]
Airway compromise less common in adults—sore throat is the most frequent complaint in adults[7]
  Gentle assessment of immunized children with mild symptoms[8]
    Mild = no cyanosis, no stridor, symptoms increase minimally with agitation[8]
Lateral neck x-ray may confirm suspicion; however, it is not necessary for the diagnosis[2,9]
  Tapering of airway (steeple sign) typical of laryngotracheitis on AP view
    Croup = barking cough, comfortable supine, normal epiglottis on visualization[2]
    Epiglottitis = anxiety, drooling, & absence of barking cough[2]
  Swollen epiglottis (thumb sign) typical of epiglottitis[10]
  Be aware of possible FB aspiration
Clinical suspicion should be high when characteristic features are present due to the possibility of complete airway obstruction[11]

Definitive diagnosis is direct visualization of the epiglottis but it should only be done in a setting where the airway can be secured
Blood culture (avoid painful procedures until airway assessed)

■ MANAGEMENT

Manage airway if an emergent airway obstruction is present[2,12]
Signs of near or total obstruction: Severe respiratory distress—cyanosis—panicking—drooling—tripod
Bag valve mask with 100% oxygen—contact anesthesiologist and ENT
If the patient cannot maintain saturations in the high 80s and is not improving—consider endotracheal intubation attempt as a second physician prepares to perform a surgical airway
If saturations are maintained in the high 80s and the patient is improving—consider airway management in a controlled setting (OR) by an anesthesiologist with ENT present[2,12]
If signs of near or total obstruction are not present—assemble airway specialists to consider airway management in a controlled setting and/or critical care monitoring[2,12]
Keep patient calm without painful procedures[12]
Humidified oxygen[12]
Empiric treatment: Ceftriaxone (or Cefotaxime) AND Vancomycin (or other antistaphylococcal medication)[13–15]
Carbapenem or quinolone is an option (with vancomycin) if penicillin or cephalosporin allergic
May wish to consult infectious disease & consider culture monitoring
May consider corticosteroids but there is limited evidence that it is beneficial[16–18]
Oxygen[1]
IVF for hydration[1]
Cautious use of racemic epinephrine—limited benefit and nebulized medications may exacerbate the condition[1,12]
Racemic epinephrine may also result in rebound effect: continuous administration may avoid the rebound effect[19]
Admit

☐ GENERAL

Approximately 90% of anterior bleeds occur at Kiesselbach's Plexus[1]
- Trauma—nose-picking—low moisture—rhinitis—chronic excoriation—anticoagulated patients—Osler-Weber-Rendu disease
- Relationship with HTN is unclear & may be incidental in HTN, though HTN may prolong bleeding[2,3]
- ETOH & steroids may increase risk[4]

Posterior bleeds more difficult to control & have more bleeding

■ EVALUATION

Assess contributing factors:
- Anticoagulation, surgery, medications (ASA, nasal steroids, cocaine), cirrhosis, trauma, history of nosebleeds

PT if the patient is anticoagulated[5,6]
- Not necessary as a routine test otherwise[5,6]

CBC if bleeding severe[7]
- Type and cross if transfusion required[7]

■ MANAGEMENT

Blow nose to clear clots

Administer nasal oxymetazoline, then have patient pinch nostrils for > 10 minutes[8]
- (this method stops bleeding in 65% of patients = unlikely to cause HTN)[8]

Consider anxiolytic: Lorazepam

If not controlled—may clear clots with suction. Inspect to identify the source of bleeding

May cauterize with silver nitrate if site identified, though it requires a relatively bloodless surface. Must achieve hemostasis first[9]

Consider topical tranexamic acid (TXA)[10]
- Soak 500 mg/5 mL: apply via gauze—leave for 20 minutes

Consider anterior packing
- Rapid Rhino works quite well—do not apply antibiotic ointment if using this product—just has to be immersed in saline for approximately 30 seconds prior to insertion—packing usually left in place for 3 days
- If bleeding persists with anterior packing—consider posterior packing

Hospitalization generally required for posterior packing[11]
  Complication rates (3%) include aspiration, MI, and hypovolemia[11]
  Potential for airway and vascular complications
ENT follow-up in 2–3 days for anterior packing.
Antibiotics are not necessary for anterior packing[10,12]
After packing is removed apply saline nasal spray 2 puffs 5 times per day for several weeks to keep the nasal mucosal surface moist (if there was no packing placed the saline nasal spray should still be used for several weeks)

STEVENS–JOHNSON SYNDROME

☐ GENERAL

Erythema multiforme (EM) is an immune-mediated, self-limited process characterized classically by target skin lesions
- It is distinctly different from Stevens–Johnson syndrome (SJS), which is a severe mucocutaneous reaction[1]

EM major = mucosal involvement (though similar to SJS—evidence suggests they may be different disorders)[1]
- SJS is typically drug induced[2]

EM minor = no mucosal involvement

EM—multiple etiologies have been described such as bacterial infections and viruses (herpes), medications especially PCN and sulfa, autoimmune, and malignancy[3]

■ EVALUATION

Mostly a clinical diagnosis[4,5]

Exam: round target lesions are the classic presentation but they are not always present[4]
- Dark red inflammatory ring—dull central area or blister—halo on the periphery—these findings make up the classic target
- Mucosal lesions if present are generally asymptomatic[3]
- Fever and body aches are more common in cases with mucosal involvement[3]
- Duration of lesions is approximately 2 weeks[4]

SJS mimics EM major[5]
- SJS lesions typically more truncal
- SJS skin tenderness is more common
- SJS exhibits more systemic symptoms, such as fever, myalgia, malaise
- SJS recent medication ingestion is more common
- SJS lesions tend to be more macular as opposed to EM having papular lesions

Labs not specific[3,4]:
- CBC (WBC may be elevated)
- Chemistries (liver enzymes may be elevated)
- ESR (may be elevated)
- Consider herpes simplex serology[6]

In general, labs are not required in most routine EM cases.
SJS: also coagulation studies, CRP, mycoplasma serology, U/A
CXR if respiratory symptoms are present

■ MANAGEMENT

Mild disease with skin or limited po mucosal involvement that is not hindering the patient who does not appear ill—no extensive RCTs to guide management except for symptomatic treatment
- Topical corticosteroids
  - Po antihistamines
  - Po formulations of lidocaine, diphenhydramine, & antacids
  - Discontinue drugs that may be the etiology

Severe po mucosal involvement
- Prednisone 40–60 mg/d then tapered over next 2–3 weeks[7]

Admit severe cases of EM especially[8]:
- Skin loss
- Inability to tolerate po

Consult ophthalmology if ocular involvement[8]

Severe widespread mucocutaneous reaction with blistering, skin sloughing, & systemic symptoms is classic SJS[9]

SJS and TEN (toxic epidermal necrolysis) are regarded by some to be similar diseases along the same spectrum that vary in severity. TEN is usually diagnosed when more than 30% of the skin surface is involved
- ICU or burn unit is the preferred treatment setting[9]
  - IVF resuscitation
  - IV immune globulin (IVIG) is typically utilized—efficacy unclear[10]
  - IV dexamethasone decreases mortality[11]

□ GENERAL

Methanol & ethylene glycol are rapidly absorbed (peak serum concentration 1–2 hours)[1]
- 1 g/kg (methanol or ethylene glycol) is considered lethal in the absence of treatment
- Product guides seldom have concentrations:
  - Generally 50% vol/vol solutions have 0.4 g/mL methanol or 0.6 g/mL ethylene glycol

Commercial products: antifreeze, automotive preparations (generally contain fluorescein), cleaners, solvents

Parent alcohols are essentially nontoxic—goal is to prevent oxidization of toxic metabolites[2]

Early toxicity: CNS depression & intoxication symptoms similar to ethanol

Late toxicity: metabolic acidosis with elevation in anion gap (osmolar gap as well), tachypnea, altered mental status

Muscle incoordination, headache, slurred speech, altered mental status, vomiting, seizure, lethargy
- Blindness, visual changes typical of methanol toxicity
- Flank pain, oliguria, and hematuria typical of ethylene toxicity

■ EVALUATION

Glucose (evaluate for hypoglycemia)

Acetaminophen & salicylate levels (evaluation for co-ingestions)

ECG (ethylene glycol can prolong the QT interval due to effects on calcium)

Chemistries (anion gap/renal function)
- Note serum osmolality

Lactate (may be elevated)[3]

Serum ethanol concentration (to help determine the osmolal gap)

Serum methanol, isopropanol, & ethylene glycol concentrations
- Do not rely on the serum tests noted above

U/A (for crystals)
- Oxalate crystal formation is a nonspecific & late finding[4]
- Fluorescein exam of urine is frequently performed, but is a poor diagnostic test with limited value[5,6]

Consider HCG
Definitive diagnosis: ethylene glycol concentration > 50 mg/dL[4]
  If it is lower you cannot rule out toxicity (parent compound may be partially metabolized)[4]
Suggestive of the diagnosis[4]:
  History of ingestion—osmolar gaps > 10 units in acute ingestion
  Unexplained anion gap metabolic acidosis after considering other causes
  Hypocalcemia

MANAGEMENT

Airway control of intoxicated patients—hyperventilate if intubated
IVF resuscitation & vasopressors if needed
Fomepizole 15 mg/kg IV load then 10 mg/kg q 1 h × 4 doses (blocks alcohol dehydrogenase)[7]
Sodium bicarb 1–2 mEq/kg bolus then 132 mEq infusion $NaHCO_3$ in 1 L D5W at 200–250 mL/h for pH < 7.3
Known methanol toxicity: give folic acid 50 mg IV q 6 h in addition to fomepizole
Known ethylene glycol toxicity: thiamine 100 mg IV & pyridoxine 50 mg IV in addition to fomepizole[8]
Consult for hemodialysis[9]
Admit: CNS depression—airway control—suicidal intent—administration of fomepizole & significant ingestions
Discharge: no suicide intent—no ethanol concentration detected with no laboratory abnormalities
Recommend calling Poison Control if any toxic alcohol ingestion is suspected

GENERAL

Classic definition: prolonged febrile illness without definite cause[1]
- Fever > 100.9°F
- Duration at least 3 weeks
- Unclear etiology after hospital evaluation

Emergency departments encounter fever where duration & degree may not yet be established
- True fever of unknown origin (FUO) is uncommon

Origin: percentages vary widely depending on the study & inclusion criteria[2]
- Infectious 20–40% (abscesses, endocarditis, tuberculosis, osteomyelitis, UTI)
- Noninfectious 10–30% (juvenile RA, lupus, temporal arteritis, polymyalgia rheumatica)
- Malignancy 20–30% (leukemia, renal cell carcinoma)
- Other 10–20% (subacute thyroiditis, drug fever, alcoholic cirrhosis)

EVALUATION

No evidence-based guidelines have been established—initial workup may include[2]:

History & physical
CBC
Chemistries
Hepatitis serologies if liver functions abnormal
Blood cultures
U/A & culture
CXR
Calcium
ESR, CRP
Procalcitonin
ANA antibodies
RA factor
Serum lactate
HIV antibody
Specific organ system eval will require specific testing & specialist consultation may be needed for complex cases[3]

MANAGEMENT

Avoid empiric management except in certain cases such as[3]:
- Antimicrobials for suspected culture-negative endocarditis
- Steroids for suspected temporal arteritis
- Antituberculosis drugs for suspected TB
- Discontinuing drugs in suspected drug fever

Neutropenic patients with fever should be treated with antimicrobials quickly & with broad spectrum[4]

Disposition dependent on the origin of fever, comorbidities, and severity of the disease

ERYTHEMA INFECTIOSUM (PARVOVIRUS B19)

☐ GENERAL

Fifth disease is characterized by a "slapped cheek" appearance—it is usually a mild febrile illness with a rash being the most common manifestation of parvovirus B19 infection[1]

Five syndromes of parvovirus B19[2]:
- Fifth disease/erythema infectiosum (most common)
- Transient aplastic crisis
- Polyarthritis
- Hydrops fetalis resulting in miscarriage
- RBC aplasia/anemia in immunocompromised patients

Person-to-person transmission is the most common (respiratory droplets)[3]

Asymptomatic or flu-like symptoms: slapped cheek rash, erythematous maculopapular truncal rash with central clearing often with a lacy appearance, and nonspecific fever, coryza, myalgia[3]

■ EVALUATION

Clinical diagnosis[3]
- Labs confined to immunocompromised patients, pregnant women, or patients with transient aplastic crisis[3]

Antibody testing for detection of immunoglobulin M confirms the diagnosis in immunocompetent patients

CBC (decreased reticulocyte count & Hgb concentration)[4]

■ MANAGEMENT

No specific treatment is necessary[3]
- Supportive management
- NSAIDs for arthralgias

Weekly ultrasound for pregnant women to monitor for hydrops fetalis[3]

Blood transfusions for transient aplastic crisis[3]

Most infections are benign, self-limited, and resolve within a few weeks[3]

34 Foreign Bodies

☐ GENERAL

Indications for removal of skin foreign body[1]:
  FB causing: pain—infection—cosmetic purposes—joint mobility dysfunction
  Organic material (highly infectious risk): wood—vegetative matter
Inert objects (metal, glass) have lower infection risk. Must weigh trauma of removal with benefit[1]
FBs near critical structures (nerves, arteries) may need removal by specialist
Most common ingested FB is a coin[2]

■ EVALUATION

Airway & breathing are the most important aspects of an ingested FB
Imaging of the suspected area even if FB felt to be radiolucent[3]
  Flat ingested objects tend to orient coronally appearing flat/round on the AP view[4]
  Flat tracheal objects tend to orient sagittally best seen on lateral projection[4]

■ MANAGEMENT

Ingested FBs that require immediate removal[3]:
  Disc battery (esophageal)
  Sharp, long (> 5 cm), or superabsorbent polymer
  Airway compromise or obstruction
  Fever, abd pain, vomiting
  Esophageal FB & > 24 hours since ingestion or unknown time
May observe[3]:
  Blunt objects
Magnet ingestion consult gastroenterologist[5]
  If it is a single magnet within the stomach there is an option of serial x-ray monitoring with "magnet precautions": avoid magnetic objects nearby
Battery ingestion: consult gastroenterology as guidelines differ & unclear which provides better outcomes[6]
  National Battery Ingestion Hotline 202-625-3333

Skin FB: see "General" above
- Weigh risk/benefit
- Fish hooks push through, cut barb then back out
- Consider incision to expose superficial FBs
- Consider wide tissue elliptical incision for deep FBs[1]

Td booster as needed

35 GI Bleed

☐ GENERAL

Most predictive finding for upper GI Bleed is melena. Most predictive finding for lower GI Bleed is clots in stool, bright red blood/maroon stools[1]
- Melena can occur with only 50 mL of blood

No evidence that NG lavage changes outcome[2]

Establish history: previous GI bleed—anticoagulation drugs—ulcer disease—cirrhosis

■ EVALUATION

Assess hemodynamic status[3–5]
- Mild hypovolemia[5]: tachycardia at rest
- Mod hypovolemia[5]: orthostatic hypotension (systolic BP decreases > 20 mmHg and/or heart rate increases > 20 beats per minute between supine and standing [15% blood loss])
- Severe hypovolemia[5]: supine hypotension (40% blood loss)

Consider endotracheal intubation in patients predisposed to aspiration or severe cases (dementia, severe bleeding, hypovolemic patients)

Labs:
- CBC
- Chemistry (include LFTs)
- PT/INR, PTT
- Blood type/cross if suspect need for transfusion
- Cardiac enzymes if MI risk
- ECG if MI risk

There is evidence that Hgb & Hct measurements drop fairly quickly in acute bleeding[6,7]
- An initial normal hemoglobin does not completely rule out significant bleeding

There is no diagnostic or therapeutic benefit from gastric lavage[8]

Rectal exam: test for melena for UGI. Examine for fissures or hemorrhoids for LGI
- Hemacult stool test

Signs of peritonitis suggest perforation

MANAGEMENT

NPO
Establish two large bore IVs (18 gauge or larger)
Infuse NS or lactated ringers (at least 500 mL over 30 minutes)[9]
Transfuse blood[10]
  Hgb < 9 g/dL in high risk (advanced age, CAD)
  Hgb < 7 g/dL in low risk
  Avoid overtransfusion of suspected variceal bleed (can make the bleed worse)[10]
    Transfuse to Hgb ≥ 10 g/dL[10]
Pantoprazole (PPI) 80 mg IV then infusion 8 mg/h[11]
  Variceal bleeding
    Octreotide 50 mcg IV bolus then infusion 50 mcg/h
  Cirrhosis patients
    Ceftriaxone 1 g/day IV
No role has been demonstrated for the use of tranexamic acid (TXA)[12]
Reverse anticoagulation on an individualized basis depending on the severity
  Vitamin K 10 mg IV over 10–20 minutes (Warfarin)
  4-Factor prothrombin complex concentrate (Kcentra)
Consult a GI Specialist
Blatchford score[13]

BUN (mg/dL)	
< 18.2	0
18.2–22.3	+2
22.4–28	+3
28–70	+4
> 70	+6

Hemoglobin (g/dL) for men	
> 13	0
12–13	+1
10–12	+3
< 10	+6

Hemoglobin (g/dL) for women	
> 12	0
10–12	+1
< 10	+6

Systolic blood pressure (mmHg)	
≥ 110	0
100–109	+1
90–99	+2
< 90	+3

Other criteria	
Pulse ≥ 100 (per minute)	+1
Melena present	+1
Presentation with syncope	+2
Liver disease history	+2
Heart failure history	+2

Any score > 0 is at high risk for intervention: transfusion, surgery
0 = low risk
Admit UGI bleed for early endoscopy
- Blatchford score may aid risk stratification of outpatient management for select patients < 60 yo with no comorbidities, hypotension, or tachycardia. The decision is usually made with GI consultation when there is easy access to outpatient endoscopy and no suspicion of having variceal bleeding[14,15]

Admit LGI bleed for early colonoscopy
- Outpatient management may be indicated in select cases of no hemodynamic compromise, no gross bleeding, age < 60 yo, or if exam reveals an anorectal source

ACUTE ANGLE CLOSURE

☐ GENERAL

Defined as optic neuropathy. Typically associated with increased intraocular pressure (IOP), but not always[1]
Second leading cause of blindness. The first leading cause is cataracts[2]
Angle closure = 1/3 of cases[3]
  Angle closure causing sudden obstruction with elevated IOP
Open angle = 2/3 of cases[3]
  Open angle is chronic and usually asymptomatic early in the disease. It is typically identified through screening
Risk factors: advanced age (> 60 yo), family history of angle closure, female, farsighted, non-Caucasian (Asians higher risk)[4]
Severe ocular pain (generally unilateral)—sudden loss of vision or blurred vision—halos around lights—headache—eye redness—nausea/vomiting—mildly dilated hazy/cloudy pupil reacting poorly to light[3]
History can be very important. Decreased light (turning lights off or walking into a dark room may trigger the process) causes papillary dilatation blocking the angle[5]
  Do not dilate eyes in the ER. Defer to ophthalmology

■ EVALUATION

Eye exam
  Gonioscopy is the gold standard for diagnosis. The ophthalmologist uses the slit lamp to visualize the angle
Evaluate IOP,[6] visual acuity, & visual field testing[7]
  Elevated IOP is the main risk factor for glaucoma but it is not sufficient alone for diagnosis[8]
    Positive predictive value 52.1%[8]
    Negative predictive value 99.4%[8]
      Normal IOP: 8–21 mmHg[8]
      Increased IOP = > 21 mmHg[8,9]
Periocular pain—N/V—blurred vision with a history of halos—conjunctival injection and/or mild mid-dilated unreactive pupil accompanies elevated IOP[10]

■ MANAGEMENT

Immediate ophthalmology consult
  Empiric treatment if the delay will be > 1 hour & suspicion is high[11]
Place patient supine: morphine/antiemetics are safe
If an hour or more delay before ophthalmology can see patient, a typical regimen may look like this but in consultation with ophthalmology[3,12]:
    Timolol maleate 0.5% 1 gtt—wait 1 min
    then
    Apraclonidine 1% 1 gtt—wait 1 min
    then
    Pilocarpine 2% 1 gtt—q 15 min for 2 total doses, wait 1 min after the 1st dose
    then
    Prednisolone acetate 1% 1 gtt q 15 min for 4 total doses
    Acetazolamide 500 mg IV (PO if IV not available)
If IOP remains significantly increased (> 40) after 30 min & ophthalmology not available: give Mannitol 1–2 g/kg IV
  If medical treatment is successful—IOP will be decreased & the symptoms will also decrease
Treatment of choice is peripheral iridotomy

☐ GENERAL

Benign headaches include:
  Sinus: actually uncommon. Nasal symptoms are also associated with migraine[1]
  Migraine: 60–70% unilateral. 30% bifrontal or global. Gradual onset
    Photophobia. N/V[1]
  Tension: bilateral. Pressure[2]
  Cluster: always unilateral. Usually begins around the eye with tearing and
    redness usually present. Pain deep & crescendos in minutes[2]
Red flags[3]:
  Focal neurologic signs, papilledema, neck stiffness, sudden onset of worst
    H/A of life, immunocompromised state, personality changes, H/A after
    trauma, H/A worse with exercise, new onset during pregnancy, > 50 yo,
    systemic signs such as fever
Sudden onset (thunderclap)[3]:
  May represent—SAH, mass, meningitis, carotid dissection, or other serious
    intracranial disease
  Immediate CT & possibly LP if no evidence of SAH
Low risk (no red flags)[3]:
  < 30 yo
  History of similar H/As with no change in pattern
  Benign H/A features
  No high-risk comorbidities
  No new concerning findings on physical exam
Though hypertensive emergency can cause H/A—HTN is not associated with
  typical migraine or tension H/A[4,5]
Eye strain is rarely a cause of H/A due to refractive error, though correction may
  improve the pain[6]
Pain intensity is not a reliable indicator of the seriousness of underlying conditions
  causing the H/A[7]

■ EVALUATION

Physical exam: Include BP, pulse, listen for bruits, palpate head/neck, evaluate
  temporal/neck arteries, examine spine/neck
  Exam should include a neurologic evaluation

Most patients without red flags or signs have no secondary cause & do not require imaging[3,8]

Ottawa SAH rule (further evaluation if 1 or more is present in nontraumatic H/A reaching maximum < 1 hour & normal neurologic exam)[9]
- 40 yo or older
- Loss of consciousness witnessed
- Neck pain or stiffness
- Onset of pain with exertion
- Thunderclap onset (instantly peaking)
- Limited neck flexion

Lumbar puncture may be indicated if[3]:
- Sudden onset but no CT evidence & SAH is suspected
- Suspicion of meningitis (neck stiffness)
- H/A triggered by exertion (cough, intercourse)
- Neurologic findings
- Papilledema
- Systemic illness (fever, rash)
- New H/A in patient with Lyme disease, HIV, cancer

CT head for sudden onset (thunderclap)[10]
- New H/As in patients > 40 yo, cancer, Lyme, or HIV may require imaging and/or LP

MRI with/without contrast may be appropriate for patients with red flag features[11]

CRP and/or ESR if temporal arteritis suspected[12]

Other lab testing as needed for certain etiologies—H/A has one of the largest differential diagnosis in medicine (> 300 causes), although most are benign with a primary cause[13]

Do not forget angle closure glaucoma in the differential, particularly when a patient enters a dark environment

MANAGEMENT

Treat underlying cause[14]

Benign idiopathic H/As consider: NSAIDs, acetaminophen

☐ GENERAL

Presentation varies. Symptoms are nonspecific[1]

Common presentations[1]:

1. Exercise intolerance
2. Fluid retention
3. Dyspnea
4. Cardiomegaly and/or dysfunction may be an ancillary fiinding
5. Orthopnea

Diagnosis can be difficult. Inquire about weight gain, medications, noncompliance, inadvertent or intentional salt intake[2] (fried foods, fast foods, frozen dinners, V-8 juice, etc.). Many products have an enormous amount of salt

Echocardiography is the diagnostic standard for identifying heart failure, usually not done in the ED unless the provider is proficient at cardiac ultrasound[3]

■ EVALUATION

CXR[4]

ECG

CBC

Chemistry (and magnesium)

U/A

Cardiac panel (troponin)

BNP (useful to distinguish acute decompensation or if diagnosis is unclear and has predictive value)[3]

■ MANAGEMENT

Oxygen (sats < 90%)[4] use a non-rebreather mask[5]

Position patient upright

Loop diuretics (Lasix 40–100 mg IV)

"May use 1" NTG paste if patient is minimally SOB

IV Nitroglycerin as a diuretic adjunct if not hypotensive (or nitroprusside if very hypertensive)

Nitroglycerin 5–10 mcg/min titrate q 5 min prn (> 120 mcg/min doses may be needed)[6]

May require increasing NTG fairly quickly to at least 60 mcg/min within 10 minutes if no hypotension

Nitroprusside 0.3 mcg/kg/min. Slowly titrate q 5 min prn. Do not exceed 10 mcg/kg/min[7]

Typically utilized in serious HTN (eg, 280/160)

May use hydralazine 10–20 mg IV for blood pressure control if hypertensive

Morphine

Dopamine or dobutamine in severe systolic dysfunction

Intubate or positive pressure ventilation (BiPAP) if significant respiratory distress or severe hypoxemia

Do not give β-blocker for acute failure and/or if pulmonary edema present

American Health Care Policy Research Admission Criteria (Healthcare Research & Quality)[8]

1. Respiratory distress
2. Hypoxia (sat < 90%)
3. Anasarca or significant edema (> 2+)
4. Syncope/hypotension (systolic < 80 mmHg)
5. New onset (no past Hx of CHF)
6. Evidence of ischemia (chest pain)
7. Inadequate social support for outpatient management
8. Failure of outpatient management
9. Concomitant acute medical illness

GENERAL

Massive hemoptysis is usually defined as life threatening when there is > 500 mL of blood over a 24-hour period[1]
- No consensus on the definition of massive amount
- Mild bleeding with good air exchange is generally managed as an outpatient

Risk for malignancy: > 50 yo, smoking history, long duration of symptoms[2,3]
< 30 mL: minor[3]
30–300 mL: moderate to severe[3]
> 300 mL: massive[3]
Type/cross blood for massive bleeding

EVALUATION

CXR (most important initial study)[4]
CBC (assess magnitude & chronicity)
Chemistries (assess for renal & liver functions)
Urinalysis (screen for pulmonary/renal syndromes)
PT/INR/PTT (assess coagulopathy as a contributing factor)
Sputum culture (case-by-case basis)
BNP (if heart failure is suspected)
D-dimer (if PE is suspected)
Pulse oximeter or ABG (assess oxygenation)
CT chest should be considered with a positive CXR for malignancy or high risk (> 40 yo or heavy smoking history)[3]
Bronchoscopy provides definitive visualization[5]

MANAGEMENT

< 30 mL blood, known or likely cause (ie, bronchitis, which is the number one cause), absent risk factors for malignancy, and normal CXR[6]
- Observe if viral bronchitis is suspected
- Treat with an antibiotic if bacterial bronchitis is suspected

> 30 mL in 24 hours without clear cause, normal CXR[6]

Bronchoscopy (CT in ER if bronchoscopy not immediately available)[7]

Bronchoscopy & CT are complementary studies[7]

Isolated streaks of blood may be managed as outpatient

> 50 yo or risk factors (smoking): levaquin and pulmonology F/U

Younger: Z-pak

Gross bleeding—admit

☐ GENERAL

Varicella-zoster virus (VZV): primary VZV is varicella (chickenpox). Reactivation of latent VZV is zoster (shingles)

Painful unilateral vesicular eruption is typically along a dermatome distribution beginning as erythematous papules[1]

- Lesions crust in 7–10 days & are no longer infectious—new lesions > 1 week suggests possible immunodeficiency [1]
- Rash + acute neuritis are typically thoracic & lumbar dermatomes—zoster keratitis/ophthalmicus may threaten vision[2,3]

Most patients (75%) have prodromal pain before rash appears with pain being the most common symptom[3]

- Pain can be produced by light touch

Maternal varicella may affect the fetus but transmission to fetus is rare[4,5]

■ EVALUATION

Exam: a dermatomal painful rash that does not cross midline[6]

- Itchy, tingling, and painful even to light touch

Diagnosis is clinical—atypical rash can be cultured for varicella zoster virus[6]

Cerebrospinal fluid analysis if there is suspected CNS involvement

■ MANAGEMENT

Best to treat immunocompetent patients < 72 hours from onset of rash

PO treatment options[6]:

- Acyclovir 800 mg 5× daily for 7 days
- Valacyclovir 1 g TID for 7 days
- Famciclovir 500 mg TID for 7 days
- If cost is not an issue use valacyclovir or famciclovir because there is less incidence of postherpetic neuralgia
- IV acyclovir for CNS, disseminated, or severely immunocompromised, ocular involvement

Pain control: NSAIDs, acetaminophen, or combination with a low potency opioid (codeine/tramadol)[1,6]

- Potent opioids should be used for severe pain[1]

Ophthalmic zoster: red eye, photophobia, tearing, vision change, lesions on the tip-of-nose [Hutchinsons's sign], or suspicion of ocular involvement: Emergent Ophthalmology Consult[7]
- Ophthalmic antimicrobial ointment—mydriatic/cycloplegia (iritis)—pressure reducing ocular drugs (glaucoma)—IV acyclovir (retinitis) may be considered

Ramsay Hunt syndrome (herpes zoster oticus) unilateral facial paralysis, ear canal vesicles, & ear pain[8]
- Facial paralysis may be more severe than Bell's palsy & typically treated with antivirals[8]
- No evidence that antiviral plus corticosteroids are more beneficial than corticosteroids alone[9]
- Consult ENT[10]

Gabapentin 300 mg qhs or 100–300 mg TID (based on postherpetic neuralgia [PHN] usage)[1] or

Nortriptyline 25 mg qhs may titrate by 25 mg/d q 2–3 days max 150 mg/d (based on PHN usage)[1]

Prednisone taper (typically: 60 mg daily for 7 days, then 30 mg daily for 7 days, then 15 mg daily for 7 days)[11]
- Combined with acyclovir improves quality of life in immunocompetent patients[10]

Post herpetic neuralgia treatment:
- Tricyclic antidepressants (nortriptyline), gabapentin, or pregabalin[12]
- Capsaicin or topical lidocaine is an option for less severe pain
- Due to abuse potential—opioids used cautiously & usually not first-line therapy[13]

☐ GENERAL

Singultus—intermittent involuntary diaphragmatic spasm & intercostal muscle spasm[1]

- Bout: duration up to 48 hours
- Persistent: duration 48 hours to 1 month
- Intractable: duration > 1 month

Mechanism unclear—80% involve unilateral contraction of left hemidiaphragm[2]

- Hiccups are typically benign and self-limited. If acute they typically last minutes to hours[3]
- Over 100 diseases and etiologies are known to induce persistent or intractable hiccups[3]

■ EVALUATION

Persistent (> 48 hours) & intractable (> 1 month) require attempts to identify cause[3,4]

- Specific cause not found in many patients[5]

Complete physical exam including neurologic exam and medication history[3]

Labs[3,4,6]:

- Usually no labs are required
- CBC
- Chemistries (BUN/creatinine, liver functions)
- Calcium
- Amylase/lipase
- ESR
- ECG (consider troponin)
- CXR

Consider other studies suggested by exam[3,4,6]:

- Usually no imaging is required
- Abdominal x-ray
- Ultrasound
- MRI head if neuro symptoms or worsening H/As
- CT chest if abnormal CXR
- LP if meningitis suspected
- Drug screen
- Endoscopy if GI findings

■ MANAGEMENT

No broad randomized trials to guide treatment—modalities based on case report[7]
First target any causative disease (GERD, MI, cancer)
Non-pharmacologic[3]:
- Vagal stimulation (apply pressure to eye, bridge of nose, upper lip)
- Stimulate uvula (sip cold water, gargling, lift uvula with spoon)
- Interfere with respiration (valsalva, holding breath)
- Counteract diaphragmic irritation (pull knees to chest, induce sneezing)
- Sexual intercourse has a case report of stopping intractable hiccups[8]

Chlorpromazine is the drug of choice[4,9]
- Only drug FDA approved for hiccups (contraindicated in the elderly with dementia)
- 25–50 mg po 3–4 times daily
- 25–50 mg IM if persistent hiccups after 3–4 days of po treatment
- 25–50 mg slow IV infusion with patient supine and BP monitoring with a 500–1000 mL saline infusion
  (if hiccups are persistent after po & IM treatment)

Baclofen has been studied as a treatment for chronic hiccups[10,11]
Metoclopramide 10 mg TID or QID[12]
- 5–10 mg IV or IM q 8 h

Gabapentin 300 mg qhs (will need to titrate up to 900 mg/d over several weeks)[13]
- Other dosing: 100 mg BID or 600 mg qhs have been reported

Dexamethasone has been used in chemotherapy patients[14]

□ GENERAL

Etiologies include trauma, pathologic, or stress fractures
Inability to walk—hip in abduction & externally rotated with leg shortening[1]
Exam may not be obvious in cognitively impaired patients[1]
Careful exam to determine the cause of fall (ie, syncope) & extent of other injuries (ie, spinal fracture)
Fracture & Mortality (FRAMO) Index is predictive of 2-year risk of mortality[2]

1. Age > 80 yo
2. Weight < 132 lbs
3. Hx of fragility fracture after 40 years
4. Need to use arms to rise from sitting (can patient rise 5 times without using arms?)

<u>2-year cumulative hip fx incidence or death</u>
0 risk factors = 2.4% mortality/0.8% hip fx
1 risk factor = 3.8% mortality/0.7% hip fx
2 risk factors = 15% mortality/5.7% hip fx
3 risk factors = 33.3% mortality/4.1% hip fx
4 risk factors = 51.5% mortality/9.1% hip fx

■ EVALUATION

Hip and pelvis x-ray is fine for most patients[1,3]
MRI is considered the test of choice if in doubt (such as patient cannot walk despite normal x-ray) as it may reveal occult fracture[1,3,4]
CT is not a routine option, though sometimes it is more available
Less reliable in determining femoral neck fractures[3]
Preoperative: (NPO for surgery)
CBC—chemistries—coag studies[5]—U/A—type and screen—CXR—ECG and other studies directed by exam & etiology of fall

■ MANAGEMENT

Adequate pain management: morphine/Hydromorphone
Pain is often undertreated in elderly & increases delirium risk[6]

Consider femoral nerve block if adequately trained with ultrasound.
Consult orthopedics
Anticipate perioperative needs: antimicrobials, oxygen, anticoag ulant reversal, Foley
Preoperative traction should not be used[7]
Surgery within 48 hours reduces mortality & risk of pressure sores[8]

GENERAL

Mild[1]: $K^+ > 5.5$–5.9 mEq/L
Mod[1]: K^+ 6–6.5 mEq/L
Severe[1]: $K^+ > 6.5$ mEq/L or ECG changes and $K^+ > 5.5$ or symptomatic & $K^+ > 5.5$ (symptoms: muscle weakness, arrhythmia, paralysis, ileus)
If no symptoms or risk factors—consider hemolyzed specimen & repeat test[2]
Seen in many conditions such as renal disease, DM, & lupus
Most have chronic hyperkalemia < 6.5 mEq/L with no symptoms & do not require rapid reduction

EVALUATION

CBC (examine for causes—leukocytosis, thrombocytosis)
Chemistry (examine renal function & for hyperglycemia)
Calcium & magnesium
ECG (examine for changes related to hyperkalemia)[3]
- Earliest change = peaked, narrow T waves & shortened QT
- K^+ concentration > 7 = widening QRS, decreased p wave amplitude

Cardiac monitoring
Urine K^+, creatinine, & osmolarity are helpful in differentiating renal from other causes but not done in the ED
Blood pH & anion gap are helpful to assess for renal tubular acidosis
Consider total CK if rhabdomyolysis is suspected
Low aldosterone levels, low cortisol, & high renin are present in adrenal insufficiency (low Na^+—high K^+)[4]
- Unexplained hyperkalemia with hypotension: consider cortisol & ACTH levels
- Then give 100 mg Hydrocortisone IV for presumed adrenal insufficiency[5]

MANAGEMENT

Indications for Tx[2,6]:
- $K^+ > 6.5$ mEq/L (6.5 mmol/L) even if no ECG changes
- OR hyperkalemia associated with ECG changes or muscle weakness or paralysis
- OR hyperkalemia with impaired renal function or significant acidosis

Calcium gluconate 10–20 mL of 10% solution over 2–3 minutes (0.5 mL/kg for peds) (repeat if needed)[7]

Utilized to stabilize the myocardium—has no effect on K^+ levels

Inhaled albuterol (shifts extracellular to intracellular space)[8]

Regular insulin 10 units plus glucose 40–60 g IV bolus (shifts from extracellular)[7]

Peds: glucose 0.5 g/kg/h plus insulin 0.05 units/kg/h if glucose > 180 mg/dL

Kayexalate (sodium polystyrene sulfonate) 15 g 1–4 times daily (slow to act = 24 h)[7]

Due to minimal K^+ effects & potential adverse effects, its use is controversial[7,8]

No sorbitol as it may be the cause of most intestinal necrosis[9]

Dialysis as a second line unless already a dialysis patient or life-threatening hyperkalemia

Sodium bicarbonate has limited/inconclusive evidence (fast acting)[2,7]

Its use is controversial[2,7,9–11]

Admit:

Severe $K^+ > 8$ with ECG changes other than peaked T waves[12]

Most ED physicians will admit patients with a $K^+ > 6$

Worsening renal function[12]

Comorbidities or medical issues requiring management[12]

Hospital admission may not change outcome based on limited (23 participants) cohort study[12]

☐ GENERAL

Severe BP elevation (> 180 mmHg systolic/> 120 mmHg diastolic) plus evidence of end-organ damage or impending complications[1]
- Limited evidence to guide hypertensive urgency management of < 180/120[1-3]
- May be more risk than benefit from aggressively lowering BP in asymptomatic patients with BP > 180/120[1-3]

HTN emergency= > 180/120 plus end-organ damage evidence[1]
HTN urgency= > 180/120 without end-organ damage evidence[1]
- It may include upper Stage II with H/A, anxiety, or dyspnea

Rate of blood pressure elevation is more important than absolute BP level[4]
Normal SBP < 120 mmHg & DBP < 80 mmHg[5]

Stage I=	140–159/90–99 (evaluation within 2 months)[5]
Stage II=	> 160–179/100–109 (evaluation within 1 month)[5]
Stage III=	> 180/> 110 (evaluation within 1 week)[5]

HTN emergency is uncommon < 2 cases per million[6]
- Eclampsia is the least common, whereas CVA & pulmonary edema are the most common[6]

■ EVALUATION

Review all Rx meds particularly antihypertensive regimen, adherence, and last dose. Often the patient's salt load/diet is a significant contributing factor
- Ask about concomitant Viagra use as nitrate administration may be fatal

Determine if the patient has[7]:
- Head injury, neurologic symptoms, end-organ damage (such as retinopathy), chest pain, or acute back pain
- Pulmonary edema, pregnancy, or drugs that can produce hyperadrenergic state (cocaine, amphetamine)—recent discontinuation of clonidine
- Consider subarachnoid hemorrhage in patients with sudden, severe H/A
- Consider CVA with focal or lateralizing symptoms
- Confirm BP in both arms generally with exam for end-organ damage
- Evaluate eye findings (retinopathy, papilledema)

Evaluate for murmurs, pulmonary edema, abdominal bruits, extremity pulses, and mental status

Labs[8]:

- CBC
- Chemistries (specifically electrolytes, BUN, creatinine)
- Toxicology if sympathetic crisis is possible
- Cardiac panel if ischemia is suspected
- U/A
- ECG
- Imaging for specific clinical presentations
  - CXR if dyspnea or CP
  - CTA chest if unequal pulses or widened mediastinum on CXR for dissecting aorta
  - CT head if head injury, n/v, or neurologic symptoms
  - Echocardiogram if there is pulmonary edema for diastolic dysfunction

■ MANAGEMENT

Insufficient evidence that pharmacologic management reduces morbidity/mortality[9]

- Cochrane: 15 RCTs' systematic review

<u>HTN Urgency</u>[1,10]:

Observe for several hours after po antihypertensive treatment to lower gradually over 24–48 hours: adjust med: confirm F/U

- Labetalol 200 mg PO then another dose after 6–12 hours if needed
- Nicardipine 20–40 mg PO q 8–12 h
- Clonidine 0.2 mg PO[11]
- Other options include captopril or hydralazine[12]

<u>HTN Emergency</u>[13]:

Admit to ICU

IVF to restore intravascular volume/organ perfusion & prevent an abrupt decrease in blood pressure

Lower BP by 10–15% 1st hour (for aortic dissection BP is lowered much more aggressively)

General:

Nicardipine infusion 5 mg/h, increase by 2.5/h q 5 min to 15 mg/h MAX

Sodium nitroprusside 0.3–0.5 mcg/kg/min, increase by 0.5 mcg/kg/min gradual to 10 mcg/kg/min MAX

Labetalol 10–20 mg IV followed by 20–80 mg at 10-min intervals until target—300 mg max cumulative dose

Specific conditions:

Dissection= target < 120 (SBP) within 10–15 minutes & HR 60 = β-blocker & vasodilator

Esmolol or **metoprolol** plus **nicardipine** or **nitroprusside**

Vasodilator use with β-blocker to prevent reflex tachycardia

Ischemic CVA= lower BP may increase ischemia in the peri-infarct area

If > 185 (SBP) or > 110 (DBP) and patient is eligible for rt-PA (thrombolysis)

Labetalol 10–20 mg IV over 1–2 minutes, may repeat once

Maintain < 180/105 for at least 24 hours after thrombolysis

For non-thrombolysis candidates = consensus is to withhold med unless SBP > 220 or DBP > 120

Hemorrhagic CVA= avoid lowering < 140 SBP during first 24 hours[14]

Options include: esmolol, hydralazine, labetalol, nitroglycerin, nicardipine

MI = nitroglycerin drug of choice

Alternatives: labetalol, esmolol, nicardipine

Pulmonary edema= requires preload/afterload reduction

Nitroglycerin or Nitroprusside

Also diuretics to reduce pulmonary congestion (Lasix) (see Chapter 38)

ARF = nicardipine (nitrates accumulate in RF pts)

HTN Encephalopathy= treat promptly—delay may lead to seizure

Lower MAP 20–25% 1st hour then target 160/90–100

Labetalol or nicardipine

Avoid nitroprusside, which may increase ICP[15]

Preeclampsia/eclampsia= No medication is officially FDA approved in pregnancy

Initiate treatment for DBP > 105–110

Labetalol or hydralazine or nifedipine

Nitroprusside & ACE inhibitors contraindicated in pregnancy

May also include magnesium sulfate for seizure prevention & IVF

Sympathetic Crisis (eg, cocaine OD)= Avoid β-blockers, it may lead to unopposed alpha stimulation & increase BP

Nicardipine—verapamil—diltiazem—phentolamine

Utilize ativan in addition to antihypertensive medication

IV Agents for HTN Mgt[1]:

Nipride: 0.3–0.5 mcg/kg/min: ↑ by 0.5 mcg/kg/min until target (max 10 mcg/kg/min)

Avoid in hepatic or renal failure. It may cause hypoxemia in COPD

Nicardipine: 5 mg/h: ↑ 2.5 mg/h every 5 minutes to max 15 mg/h. Once the target is reached, wean to 3 mg/h as tolerated

Nitroglycerin: Initial 5 mcg/min: ↑ by 5 mcg/min every 3–5 minutes to 20 mcg/min; ↑ by 10 mcg/min every 5 minutes ok if

20 mcg/min is inadequate (max 200 mcg/min)—only for CHF, MI, or cardiac ischemia—NTG is not a great blood pressure reduction agent

Hydralazine (not FDA approved for HTN emergency)

10–20 mg IV bolus q 4–6 h or 10–40 mg IM

Labetalol: 20 mg IV followed by 20–80 mg boluses at 10-minute intervals until the target is achieved (max cumulative dose 300 mg)

Infusion = 0.5–2 mg/min adjusted until the target is achieved

Lopressor: 5 mg IV q 5 min × 3 (keep HR > 50–60)

Esmolol: initial load 500 mcg/kg/min over 1 minute, then 50–100 mcg/kg/min: titrate q 4 min

To increase = repeat bolus dose & increase infusion 50 mg/kg/min increments to max 200 mg/kg/min

Po Agents[11]:

Clonidine: (onset 30–60 minutes) 0.1–0.2 mg

Labetalol: (onset 20 minutes–2 hours) initial 200 mg, then repeat in 6 hours

☐ GENERAL

Reference ranges may vary but it is generally defined as potassium < 3.6 mEq/L[1]
- May become symptomatic < 2.5–3.0 mEq/L[1]
- Mild 3.1–3.5
- Mod 2.5–3
- Severe < 2.5 (ascending paralysis & respiratory changes can occur < 2 mEq/L)

Most common etiology is due to unreplaced fluid loss such as diuretic use, vomiting, and diarrhea[2]

Duration & degree of hypokalemia are proportionate to symptoms
- Slow duration may require lower level for symptoms to occur
- Rapid decline may result in symptoms sooner

Symptoms include: muscle weakness, rhabdomyolysis, cramps, myoglobinuria, cardiac arrhythmias[3]
- May be associated with magnesium depletion as well

■ EVALUATION

Search for etiology (history/labs)

Check BP[1,2]

Chemistry
- Factitious hypokalemia may occur with elevated WBC in acute leukemia if blood is left at room temperature[4]
- Every 0.3 mEq/L decrease in serum K^+ = about 100 mEq total body K^+ deficit[5]

Magnesium

Consider ABG or bicarb levels

ECG (monitor if prolonged QT or other changes and risks)[2]

■ MANAGEMENT

Treat underlying cause of potassium loss

Replace magnesium if necessary

Dietary replacement of K^+ may be sufficient if > 3 mEq/L & asymptomatic with no cardiac disease[2]

May need K^+ if < 3.5 mEq/L and symptomatic

May need K^+ if < 4 mEq/L in HTN, heart failure, or arrhythmias
- 40–100 mEq/d PO in divided doses may be adequate
- IV replacement requires admission
  - Unable to tolerate po K^+ or in severe symptomatic hypokalemia
  - Most commonly needed in DKA–hyperglycemia conditions[6]
    - K^+ may be normal at presentation & supplement may begin at just < 4.5 mEq/L[6]
    - **Insulin therapy should be delayed until K^+ > 3.3 mEq/L to avoid complications**
    - Max IV rate 10–20 mEq/h[7]
    - Continuous monitoring with IV administration[8]

Potassium chloride is preferred formulation[9]
- Patients are often chloride depleted & raises K^+ faster than potassium bicarbonate[10]
- Consider potassium bicarbonate in metabolic acidosis

Potassium sparing diuretic can be combined with a potassium supplement with close potassium monitoring

□ GENERAL

Honey-colored crusted lesions—superficial lesion, blisters rupture causing crust
Risk factors: children 2–5 yo, crowding, poor hygiene, underlying scabies[1]
Group A strep & staph aureus—typically mixtures of both[2]
Most common in summer spread by autoinoculation

■ EVALUATION

Clinical diagnosis (can confirm by Gram stain or culture but rarely needed)
Three appearances (thin crusts key characteristic in all)
- Non-bullous: honey-colored crusted (papules, pustules, or vesicles rupture forming crusts)[3]
- Bullous: fluid-filled bullae that rupture resulting in thin brown crust[3]
- Ecthyma: crusted punched out lesions into the dermis. Raised borders[4]

■ MANAGEMENT

Topical therapy is the primary approach[4]
Po therapy for numerous lesions & always for ecthyma[4]
Topical tx:
- Bactroban ointment TID × 5 days[4]
- (retapamulin ointment is an option— BID × 5 days < 2% BSA children > 9 months old)[4]

Po tx (7-day course):
- Dicloxacillin 250–500 mg QID (children 25 mg/kg/d divided QID)[4]
- Cephalexin 250–500 mg QID (children 25 mg/kg/d divided QID)[3,4]

If MRSA suspected:
- Clindamycin 300 mg QID (children 20 mg/kg/d PO divided TID)[4]
- Trimethoprim/sulfamethoxazole BID (children 8–12 mg/kg/d [TMP] PO divided BID)[4]
- Doxycycline 100 mg PO BID (< 8 yo not recommended)[4]

Contact precautions until 24 hours after onset of antimicrobial therapy[5]
- May return to school 24 hours after treatment begins (cover-draining lesions)[5,6]
- Some schools may have 48-hour policies[6]

Clean crusts—wash hands
Usually resolves within 2 weeks with or without treatment[3]
- Ecthyma may persist for weeks & heal with scars[3]

47 Inflammatory Bowel Disease

ULCERATIVE COLITIS (UC)/CROHN'S DISEASE (CD)

☐ GENERAL

UC mild: no signs of toxicity, < 4 stools daily with or without blood, normal ESR, mild crampy abdominal pain[1]
UC moderate: > 4 loose bloody stools daily, mild anemia, no toxicity, no severe abdominal pain[1]
UC severe: > 6 loose bloody stools daily, severe abdominal cramps, fever, tachycardia > 90 minutes, anemia, elevated ESR[1]
UC occurs any age—peak age 10 to 40 yo—more common in the Caucasian than non-Caucasian demographic[2]
CD has similar demographics
UC typical symptoms include the following: bloody diarrhea, tenesmus over several weeks, fever, abdominal cramping, possible constipation[3]
CD: Abdominal cramping—chronic diarrhea > 4 weeks with or without blood and mucus—constitutional symptoms such as
fever, weight loss, fatigue (may use Crohn's Disease Activity Index [CDAI])
CD: suspect if there is chronic diarrhea, weight loss, anemia, & evidence of inflammation (increased ESR/CRP)

■ EVALUATION

History & physical
Note: NSAID use & recent antimicrobial use (C. diff suspicion)[4]
CBC
Chemistries (liver functions)
ESR/CRP[5] (helps differentiate active colitis from functional disorder)
Stool for c. difficile & routine cultures
Consider imaging studies (ultrasound, CT)[6]
Plain abdominal film may be used if perforation suspected
In CD, assess for evidence of malabsorption: electrolytes, ferritin, albumin, magnesium, calcium
Colonoscopy is the definitive study for both UC & CD

MANAGEMENT

Ulcerative proctitis: topical 5-aminosalicylic acid (5-ASA) rectally is the first-line treatment[7]
- Rectal mesalamine 1 g suppository rectally BID (po formulation is an option)

Left-sided colitis (UC): combination po 5-ASA (sulfasalazine) and rectal 5-ASA or steroid suppositories[8]
- Po mesalazine typically requires 2–4 weeks[9]

CD: options include—
- Prednisone 40 mg daily for 1 week, then tapering dose[10]

Azathioprine 2–3 mg/kg/d (remission maintenance or to reduce steroid use)
- 5-ASA—use in CD is controversial (sulfasalazine plus steroid not shown to be superior to steroid alone)

and[11]:

Metronidazole

Ciprofloxacin
- Rifaximin & clarithromycin have also been studied with some response

Admit in case of severe disease for colonoscopy, IVFs, and steroids[4]

48 Intussusception

GENERAL

A common abdominal emergency in children aged 3 months to 3 yo, more frequently in males with typically an unknown cause[1]
- Uncommon in adults—typically a pathologic cause if found in adults[2]
- Rare in infants < 2 months[1]

Abdominal pain is the most common complaint for all ages[3]
- Age < 12 months the strongest indicators are irritability, emesis, and blood in stool[3]
- Exam may be normal between painful episodes—often confused with gastroenteritis[4]
- Lethargy may develop—often confused with meningoencephalitis[4]
  - Lethargy may be the result of endogenous opioid production[5]

EVALUATION

Exam[1,6]: Sudden intermittent abdominal pain (every 10–15 minutes)
- Ill-defined right-sided abdominal mass may be palpated
- Blood or mucus in stools ("currant jelly" stools)
- May have bilious vomiting or lethargy

Abdominal ultrasound is the preferred modality with 100% sensitivity & specificity[1,7,8]
- An x-ray may detect intussusception but cannot rule it out[1,9]
- Contrast enema may detect and treat simultaneously[1]
- CT abdomen/pelvis can detect & may identify etiology[10]
  - Less optimal as sedation may be necessary & radiation exposure is greater[10]

Lab studies are not specifically helpful but typically a CBC and chemistry may assess for dehydration

MANAGEMENT

Aggressive fluid resuscitation[1]
Barium enema is the treatment of choice
Immediate surgical consultation[1,11]

GENERAL

Systemic vasculitis typically affecting age < 5 yo—most prominent etiology of acquired coronary artery disease in childhood[1]

Clinical diagnosis: fever > 5 days & 4 out of the 5 findings below are present (incomplete disease has 2–3 of these findings)[1,2]:

- Bilateral conjunctival injection
- Cervical lymphadenopathy
- Po changes (erythematous lips & strawberry tongue)
- Extremity changes (palmer erythema & sole desquamation)
- Polymorphic rash

EVALUATION

Clinical evidence of systemic inflammation/vasculitis[3]

- CRP/ESR elevation
- CBC (thrombocytosis development usually after 1 week, leukocytosis, & anemia)
- Chemistry (hyponatremia possible—elevation in liver function tests)
- Ferritin elevation
- U/A (WBCs on microscopy—leukocyte esterase may be negative as it is not polymorphonuclear)[4]

Immediate cardiac echo at diagnosis[5,6]

Consider ECG[5]

MANAGEMENT

Immune globulin (IVIG) 2 g/kg IV infusion over 8–12 hours[7]

Aspirin (ASA) 30–100 mg/kg daily divided into 4 doses[8,9]

- IVIG with ASA reduces the coronary artery (CA) aneurysm risk[8,9]
  - CA aneurysm risk seems dependent on IVIG dose—not ASA dosing[10]
- ASA typically switched to 3–5 mg/kg per day once fever is absent 48 hours
- Avoid concomitant ibuprofen use during ASA treatment[6]

Corticosteroids possibly beneficial[11,12]

- May reduce length of stay & coronary abnormalities[11,12]

Admit & consult pediatrician/pediatric cardiology[5]

This is a disease with significant morbidity and mortality—better to over diagnose than miss this disease

50 Kidney Stone

☐ GENERAL

Calcium (mostly Ca^{++} oxalate & less often Ca^{++} phosphate) is the composition of 80% of stones[1]

Other types include uric acid, struvite, & cystine

Stones up to 4 mm - 95% pass < 40 days. Stones 5–10 mm 47% pass[2]

Mean time of passage: < 2 mm = 8 days. 2–4 mm = 12 days. > 4 mm = 22 days[3]

Risk factors: urinary composition (low volume, high calcium, high pH)

Diet (low fluid intake, low Ca^{++} diet, high oxalate, high Na^{+}, low K^{+}, high vitamin C, high sucrose/fructose)

Medical conditions (DM, gout, hyperparathyroidism, IBS)

Individual & family history of stones[4]

DASH diet (Dietary Approaches to Stop Hypertension) shown to decrease the incidence of stones[5]

Pain typically is severe, often described as crampy and intermittent. Originates in flank radiating to lower abdomen or groin (ensure to differentiate from torsion). Often there is an associated microscopic hematuria. Pain is usually not improved by sitting still

Hematuria is not detected in 10–30% of documented nephrolithiasis[6]

Ddx: pyelonephritis—ectopic pregnancy—ovarian torsion—AAA—appendicitis—obstruction—biliary colic—mesenteric ischemia—herpes zoster—malingering drug diversion patients (most differentiated via U/A & CT)

■ EVALUATION

Non-contrasted CT (stone chaser) is the image of choice[7]

Screen potentially pregnant females before imaging

U/S is the preferred imaging if pregnant or in children or in patients with prior radiation

Urinalysis—the only lab test that is mandatory

Parathyroid hormone (PTH) if primary hyperparathyroidism is suspected[8]

Electrolytes & creatinine recommended if suspicion of reduced renal function[9]

For high risk of hemorrhage, thrombocytopenia, anemia or infection: CBC[9]

Results[10]:

Creatinine elevation in dehydration & obstructive calculi
PTH & calcium elevation in hyperparathyroidism
Hypokalemia & hyperchloremia in renal tubular acidosis
Leukocytosis in infectious process or struvite calculi

STONE score[11]

Male=	2 points
Duration 6–24 hours=	1 point
Duration < 6 hours=	3 points
Nonblack race=	3 points
Nausea=	1 point
Vomiting=	2 points
Hematuria=	3 points

Risk of stone

Low=	0–5 points
Medium=	6–9 points
High=	10–13 points

MANAGEMENT

Urgent urology consultation for urosepsis
Acute kidney injury—anuria—uncontrolled pain/nausea/vomiting[12]
Pain control: NSAIDs as effective as opiates[13,14]
Opiate/NSAID combination more effective than monotherapy[15]
Toradol 30 mg IV drug of choice (1st option if creatinine is normal)
Morphine/dilaudid (combination with NSAID more effective than monotherapy)
IV acetaminophen

If slight UTI: provide antimicrobial coverage, may D/C with urology consultation—if urosepsis, admit and for possible stenting

Tamulosin 0.4 mg daily 1–2 weeks. Discontinue after expulsion. Stones > 10 mm excluded from studies[16]

Nifedipine (Ca^{++} channel blocker) is another option (tamsulosin had a better response in the studies) 10-30 mg TID up to 4 weeks or until expulsion[17]

IV hydration = No evidence of pain reduction or stone passage compared with no maintenance fluids[18]

Sexual activity > 3 times a week has shorter expulsion rate time than tamsulosin[19]
- Expulsion rate at 2 weeks (no significant difference at 4 weeks)
  - 83.9% sex
  - 47.6% tamsulosin
  - 34.8% symptomatic management

Outpatient if able to tolerate po

Admit for uncontrollable pain, fever, unable to tolerate po

Follow-up 1–14 days to check stone position & hydronephrosis[2]

Laceration Management

☐ GENERAL

Closure considerations: location, patient comorbidities, mechanism of injury, extensiveness of wound, infection risk, and cosmetic considerations
- Assess for foreign body, neuro/vascular compromise, tendon injury, and Td immunization status
- Optimal time from injury to repair not clearly defined in simple lacerations[1]
- No evidence to support wound age affects infection rate in simple lacerations[2]
- Clean wounds in healthy patients generally safe to suture up to 18 hours—hands up to 12 hours—facial wounds up to 24 hours[3]
- Relative contraindications: animal bites in non-cosmetic areas, deep punctures, non-hemostatic wounds, superficial wounds where suturing may actually increase scar formation & infection risk
- Clean gloves are as good as sterile gloves for suturing low-risk lacerations[4]
- Clean tap water is fine for wound cleansing[5]
- Tissue adhesives comparable to sutures regarding infection risk, dehiscence rates, and cosmetic results in areas not under high skin tension[6,7]
- Uncomplicated hand lacerations < 2 cm, < 8 hours old, & hemostatic after 15 minutes direct pressure with no neurovascular deficits, tendon or bone injury, and not involving nail bed have the same cosmetic outcome with less pain & less treatment time in ER (14 minutes shorter) if not sutured[8]
- Most tongue lacerations are not improved by suturing particularly in children, specifically < 1 cm, non-gaping, or determined to be minor[9,10]

■ EVALUATION

Explore for FB & internal damage, such as tendon or neurovascular injury requiring orthopedic management

Assess systemic influences on wound healing: renal insufficiency, DM, immunocompromised status, steroid use, antiplatelet drugs, or disorders of collagen synthesis such as Ehlers–Danlos

■ MANAGEMENT

Consider topical anesthetic in children[1]

Wound irrigation, foreign body (FB) removal, and devitalized tissue debridement

Tissue adhesives are used for low skin tension areas such as child facial lacerations

Staples are often used in the scalp or long trunk lacerations
Suturing is the most common repair method
Absorbable sutures for external child lacerations has been successful[3]
Routine antimicrobial prophylaxis is not recommended[11]
Antimicrobial prophylaxis is best for animal or human bites (Amoxicillin w/clavulanic acid), intraoral lacerations, open fractures, & exposed joints/tendons[11] (doxycycline or trimethoprim/sulfamethoxazole if PCN allergic)
Consult: severe contaminated wounds—large defects best suited for surgery—tendon/nerve/vascular damage requiring surgery—open fractures/joint penetrations/amputations—severe crush injury—deep hand/foot wound—full-thickness eyelid and possibly lip or ear[1]

□ GENERAL

Vaccine—preventable & highly contagious viral illness characterized by fever, rash, cough, coryza, conjunctivitis, and malaise
Incubation period 6–21 days (average 13–14 days) to rash onset[1,2]
  10–12 days to fever onset[1,2]
  Transmission typically among unimmunized patients but reported among immunized as well[3]
  Live virus reported up to 2 hours in airspace after aerosolized droplets (cough/sneeze)
  Infectious 4 days prior and 4 days after rash[2]
Suspect measles: fever, maculopapular rash, cough, coryza, conjunctivitis, and potential exposure

■ EVALUATION

Fever (may be high > 103°F), coryza, cough, conjunctivitis[2]
  Koplik spots (small blue-white spots on bright red background is pathognomonic)[2,4]
  Maculopapular rash 2–4 days after fever onset—may become confluent or petechiae[2,5]
    Blanching rash early in course—palms rarely involved[5]
CBC (thrombocytopenia, leukopenia may occur)[6]
CXR (for interstitial pneumonitis)
IgM antibodies (most common test)[7]
  Presence of IgM diagnostic though may be undetectable < 4 days of rash—persists 1–2 months[7]
  Rise (4×) of IgG[7]
Confirmatory testing through public health (CDC/Health Dept)
Detection of measles virus RNA by reverse transcription polymerase chain reaction (RT-PCR)[8]
Consider rubella, roseola, fifth disease, scarlet fever, & less common RMSF, Epstein–Barr mononucleosis, kawasaki, cytomegalovirus, staphylococcal toxic shock syndrome[9]

MANAGEMENT

Supportive care
- Diarrhea most common complication[10]
- Pneumonia most common cause of measles-related death[10]
- Encephalitis occurs in 1 per 1000 measles cases[10]
- Pregnancy-associated measles increases complications[11]

Isolate patient

Vitamin A administration has been utilized[12]

Antibiotics if a specific bacterial infection is identified[2]

☐ GENERAL

Must be distinguished from preseptal cellulitis, which is anterior to the orbital septum[1]
- No ocular signs
- Eyelid swelling anterior to orbital septum
- May be non-tender

Orbital cellulitis[2,3]
- Swelling posterior to orbital septum includes fat & ocular muscles
- May be associated with ocular signs (limited EOM, vision changes)

High risk of intracranial communication of infection[3]

Both preseptal cellulitis & orbital cellulitis may cause ocular pain & lid swelling[1,4]

Only orbital cellulitis causes involvement of extraocular muscles & tissue resulting in pain with eye movement[1,4]
- Orbital cellulitis is also more likely to have associated fever

■ EVALUATION

CT orbits with IV contrast can distinguish preseptal from orbital cellulitis[5,6]
- Indicated if necessary to differentiate extent of infection
- Edema can sometimes prevent a sufficient exam
- Look for vision changes or pain with eye movement
- Look for CNS symptoms
- If concerning for orbital cellulitis order CBC and chemistry

■ MANAGEMENT

Admit suspected orbital cellulitis for IV antimicrobials & ophthalmology consultation[7]
- Clindamycin 40 mg/kg/d IV divided q 6–8 h

Adjunct corticosteroids may reduce pain and edema[8]

54 Organophosphate

CHOLINERGIC TOXICITY

☐ GENERAL

Also see Chapter 76 General approach/Contact Poison Control Center
Cholinergic toxicity caused by organophosphates (OP), carbamates, nicotine, physostigmine, and edrophonium[1]
- Exposure: cutaneous, inhalation, or ingestion

Symptoms: Salivation, Lacrimation, Urination, Defecation, GI Dysfunction, Emesis (SLUDGE)[1]
- Miosis, bradycardia, nasal hyperemia, hypotension, flaccid paralysis
- Tachycardia & respiratory paralysis may occur with nicotine hyperstimulation

OP toxicity can create neurologic disorders 24–96 hours postexposure[2]
- Neck flexion weakness, CN abnormalities, diminished DTRs, proximal muscle weakness, and respiratory compromise

■ EVALUATION

The diagnosis is clinical as excessive cholinergic symptoms without known exposure indicate possible toxicity
- Many organophosphates have a garlic or petroleum odor

Direct measure of RBC acetylcholinesterase (RBC AChE) measures the degree of toxicity[3]
- Plasma cholinesterase activity is easier but does not correlate with the degree of toxicity[3]
- Both tests may not be readily available by most labs

Assess for myocardial ischemia (ECG/troponin)

■ MANAGEMENT

Remove contaminated clothing in a well-ventilated area to prevent exposure to health care workers
Avoid succinylcholine if intubation is required in OP toxicity
- Leads to exaggerated neuromuscular blockade as succinylcholine is metabolized by acetylcholinesterase
- Non-depolarizing drugs can be utilized (Rocuronium) but may require increase dosage due to competitive inhibition

IVF resuscitation especially if there are bradycardia and hypotension present.

- IV Atropine is the drug of choice[4]
  - Competes with acetylcholine receptors (not effective for nicotinic poisoning/ does not bind nicotinic receptors)
  - 2–5 mg IV adults
  - 0.05 mg/kg IV children
  - If no effect, the dose may be doubled every 3–5 minutes until symptoms alleviated (specifically bronchospasm/bronchorrhea)[4,5]
  - Mild-moderate cases: 2 mg q 5 min[3]
  - Severe cases: 2–6 mg with repeat doses q 2-60 minutes[4]
    - Tachycardia is not a reliable indicator of improvement & may result from hypoxia, sympathetic stimulation, or hypovolemia[5]
  - High doses (bolus or infusion) may be required[5]
- Pralidoxime may be administered along with atropine[1]
  - Reactivates acetylcholine esterase
  - It should not be used without concurrent atropine to prevent transient oxime-induced acetylcholinesterase inhibition to prevent worsening symptoms[6]
  - Treats both muscarinic & nicotinic symptoms[7]
  - 1–2 g IV slow infusion over 30 minutes for adults followed by 500 mg/h infusion
  - Rapid administration has been associated with cardiac arrest—slow infusion prevents muscle weakness[8]
    - 30 mg/kg adult bolus[9]
      - Then 8 mg/kg/h infusion adults[10]
    - 25–50 mg/kg children bolus[7] Then 10–20 mg/kg/h infusion children[10]
- Consider diazepam 5–20 mg IV for seizures, fasciculations, or anxiety[1]
  - Prophylactic doses were shown to decrease neurocognitive dysfunction[11]
- Consider phenobarbital for recurrent seizures[12,13]
  - No evidence that phenytoin has an effect on OP-induced seizures & is not recommended[12,13]
- Little evidence that activated charcoal is effective after 1 hour of ingestion[14]

55 Pancreatitis

☐ GENERAL

Atlanta criteria definition for pancreatitis[1]:
- Mild: absence of organ failure & local or systemic complications[1]
- Moderate: transient organ failure resolving in < 48 hours. Local or systemic complications without persistent organ failure[1]
- Severe: persistent organ failure > 48 hours. Cannot distinguish between moderate to severe & severe to acute in first 48 hours[1]

Suspect chronic pancreatitis in recurrent acute pancreatitis, constant abdominal pain, complications (pseudocyst, calcifications), evidence of pancreatic exocrine insufficiency (DM, maldigestion)[2]

Acute severe & persistent epigastric pain typical[3]
- Gallstone etiology onset is rapid
- Metabolic or ETOH etiology less abrupt and pain poorly localized
  - Other causes include but not limited to hyperlipidemia, trauma, medications, infection, and medical procedures
- Radiation to back in 50% of cases—N/V in 90% of cases[4]

Diagnosis of acute pancreatitis requires 2 or more criteria established within 48 hours of admission[1,5]:
- Abdominal pain consistent with pancreatitis
- Amylase and/or lipase > 3 times upper limit of normal
- Characteristic imaging findings

■ EVALUATION

Physical findings dependent on severity
- Epigastric tenderness
- May have abdominal distention and hypoactive bowel sounds due to an ileus
- Scleral icterus from obstructive jaundice if choledocholithiasis present
- Severe: fever—hypoxemia—tachypnea—hypotension
- Ecchymotic discoloration occurs in 3% of cases from hemoperitoneum[6,7]:
  - Periumbilical (Cullen's sign)
  - Flank (Grey Turner sign)

Labs[8–10]:
- Amylase[9,10] (rises 6–12 hours after onset—half-life 10 hours)
  - Due to short half-life, diagnosis may be missed in cases presenting > 24 hours from onset[9,10]

Lipase[9,10] (rises 4–8 hours after onset—peaks at 24 hours)
Elevations occur earlier—last longer than amylase[9,10]
Lipase/amylase ratio > 2 may differentiate nonalcoholic from alcoholic[11]
Ratio > 2 suggests alcoholic etiology (high lipase is typical)
Ratio < 2 suggests nonalcoholic etiology (high amylase is typical)
CBC
Chemistries (BUN, creatinine, liver functions)
ALT > 150 U/L may suggest gallstone etiology[12]
Calcium
Albumin
HCG (childbearing age women)
ABGs (if indicated for comorbidities & symptoms)
Abdominal ultrasound in acute pancreatitis
CT abdomen/pelvis (if uncertain diagnosis)
Abd x-ray (ileus)
CXR (one-third have CXR abnormalities)[13]
Though lipase & amylase are useful to diagnose pancreatitis—they cannot predict severity
APACHE II & SIRS scores can assess severity, prognosis, & guide management[14]

MANAGEMENT

Initial: fluid resuscitation & pain control
Normal saline or lactated ringers (LR) 5–10 mL/kg/h[15]
20 mL/kg over 30 minutes followed by 3 mL/kg/h if volume depleted[15]
In rare cases of hypercalcemia—LR contraindicated due to calcium content[15]
LR may reduce the incidence of SIRS compared with normal saline[16]
Opioids for pain control are effective[17]
Hydromorphone IV
Morphine IV
No evidence morphine exacerbates pancreatitis[18]
Antibiotics only if an extrapancreatic infection is suspected as infections increase mortality[19]
Prophylactic antibiotics not recommended[19]
For suspected infected necrosis—options[20]:
Imipenem–cilastatin 500 mg IV q 8 h

Meropenem 1 g q 8 h
Ciprofloxacin 400 mg IV q 12 h plus metronidazole 500 mg IV q 8 h
Insulin may be temporarily needed in some cases
Indications for monitored or ICU care[21]:
HR < 40 or > 150/min
Systolic BP < 80 mm Hg or diastolic > 120 mm Hg
Respiratory rate > 35/min
PaO_2 < 50 mm Hg
pH < 7.1 or > 7.7
Serum K^+ < 2.0 mmol/L or > 7.0 mmol/L
Serum Na^+ < 110 mmol/L or > 170 mmol/L
Serum glucose > 800 mg/dL
Serum Ca^{++} > 15 mg/dL
Anuria
Coma
Consider transfer to monitored bed or ICU for[21]:
APACHE II score > 8 (first 24 hours of admission)
Persistent SIRS (> 48 hours)
Hematocrit > 44%
BUN > 20 mg/dL
Creatinine > 1.8 mg/dL
Age > 60 yo
Comorbidities, such as cardiac or pulmonary disease, obesity

GENERAL

Peritonsillar abscess (PTA) is the most common deep neck infection with a collection of purulence[1,2]
- Sore throat (usually worse unilaterally), peritonsillar bulge, dysphagia, trismus, uvular deviation, muffled voice
- Bilateral PTA is rare[3]

Peritonsillar cellulitis is an inflammatory reaction caused by infection without an associated purulent collection

Diagnosis can be made clinically particularly with deviation of uvula & medial displacement of tonsil

EVALUATION

Assess the degree of airway obstruction
- Anxious, drooling, posturing, sick patients require close monitoring

Trismus is present in about two-thirds of cases due to the involvement of the internal pterygoid muscle[4]
- The patient may also have ear pain on the affected side

Imaging not specifically necessary to make the diagnosis of PTA

Imaging if unclear diagnosis[2]
- CT with contrast useful if infection is suspected to have spread beyond the peritonsillar space[5,6]
- Ultrasound may be sufficient to differentiate PTA from cellulitis[5,6]
- MRI is an alternative without radiation exposure[5,6]
- Smartphone-based thermal imaging with asymmetric hotspots may be useful[7]

Labs are not required to make the diagnosis[8]

Labs to support diagnosis & assess hydration[5]:
- CBC
- Chemistries
- CRP
- Consider monospot (Epstein–Barr virus IgM)
- Strep culture

Routine culture of aspirate indicated only in select cases[9]
- Recurrent
- DM
- Immunocompromised

MANAGEMENT

- Surgical intervention is promptly needed for airway compromise, enlarging mass, & significant comorbidities/complications[5,8]
- Drainage & antimicrobial management is the primary treatment[2,10]
  - Consult an ENT for drainage & individual management, as there is a spectrum of severity
  - Trial of antimicrobials is acceptable for probable cellulitis[11]
  - Abscesses < 1 cm without a muffled voice, trismus or drooling—ENT may defer drainage[5]
- IVF hydration if limited po intake[4]
- Consider outpatient management in uncomplicated cases if accepted follow-up protocol is available[5,10,12]
  - Optimal initial management is unclear & dependent on the certainty of diagnosis of PTA versus cellulitis[13]
- Inpatient indicated for[5,10]:
  - Consider for children aged < 4 yo[12]
  - Consider for age > 40 yo (risk of complications)
  - Sepsis
  - Dehydration
  - Concern for airway compromise
  - Immunocompromised or comorbidities (DM)
  - Outpatient management failure
- Admission for 24 hours of hydration & antimicrobials reserving drainage for cases unresponsive to treatment—studied successfully among children with 50% response rate to medical management[14,15]
- Topical anesthetic to control pain during drainage typically performed by ENT.[10]
  - Consider narcotics or ketorolac IV[14]
- Clindamycin (13 mg/kg per dose—max 900 mg single dose) q 8 h for children or 600 mg q 6–8 h adults IV[10]
- Ampicillin–sulbactam (50 mg/kg per dose—max 3 g single dose) q 6 h children or 3 g q 6 h adults IV[10]

If clinically improved & afebrile after IV treatment—14-days po (course < 10 days there is a risk of recurrence)[16]
- Amoxicillin-clavulanate (45 mg/kg per dose—max 875 mg) q 12 h children or 875 mg q 12 h adults
- Clindamycin (10 mg/kg per dose—max 600 mg) q 8 h children or 300–450 mg q 6 h adults

The evidence concerning the benefit of glucocorticoids is inconsistent, but may improve clinical outcomes[17,18]
- Dexamethasone 10 mg IV/IM[11]
- Methylprednisolone 2–3 mg/kg (250 mg max) IV/IM[11]

Observe several hours after drainage[11,19]
- Outpatient cases require close follow-up with strict return instructions

57 Pneumonia

☐ GENERAL

Clinical symptoms (cough, fever, tachycardia, crackles) do not have a sensitivity > 50% for clinical diagnosis using CXR as the standard[1]

Fever is noted in 80% of the cases, though it can be absent in the elderly[2]

Respiratory rate > 24/min in 45–70% & tachypnea is a sensitive sign in the elderly along with tachycardia[2]

One-third of the patients have no consolidation on CXR[2]

Definitive combination of symptoms predicting pneumonia are not clearly defined[2]

■ EVALUATION

History should determine the immune status & pathogen exposures[3]

Physical exam may find fever, tachypnea, and tachycardia[3]

Infiltrate on CXR is required for definitive diagnosis[4]

Studies[3]:
- CXR (or CT)
- CBC
- Chem 7
- CRP, procalcitonin, blood cultures, and sputum cultures are usually not ordered by ED physicians but rather the admitting physician
- Some evidence that biomarkers such as procalcitonin & CRP have some value differentiating asthma & COPD from pneumonia and viral from bacterial etiologies[5–7]
- Blood cultures for ICU patients recommended (optional for floor patients)
  - Positive culture rate is low—false positive culture rate high—positive cultures rarely modify tx[8]
- Sputum Gram stain & culture for hospitalized patients not ordered by ED provider
- Influenza A & B during outbreaks

CURB-65 score:
- 5 Variables—1 point each[9]
  1. Confusion
  2. BUN (> 19 mg/dL)
  3. Resp rate (≥ 30)

4. BP (systolic < 90 or diastolic ≤ 60)
5. Age (≥ 65 yo)

Score 0–1 = consider outpatient: 2 = consider admit: 3–5 = admit/possible ICU[9]

Pneumonia Severity Index is also a valid scoring system but less simple than CURB-65

■ MANAGEMENT

Outpatient[4]:

Previously healthy with no antimicrobial use in prior 3 months

Macrolide (azithromycin or clarithromycin) or

Doxycycline

Comorbidities

Fluoroquinolone (levofloxacin, gemifloxacin, moxifloxacin) or

β-lactam (high-dose amoxicillin, amoxicillin/clavulanic acid, cefpodoxime, or cefuroxime) PLUS a macrolide (azithromycin or clarithromycin)

Inpatient[4]:

Levaquin 500–750 mg IV or avelox 400 mg IV (bioavailability IV equal to PO) or

β-lactam plus macrolide

Inpatient nursing home acquired and/or pseudomonas concern: piperacillin-tazobactam plus Levofloxacin

Hospitalization considerations

Ability to maintain po intake, compliance, substance abuse history, mental illness, cognition, functionality, living situation

58 Preeclampsia

☐ GENERAL

Systolic > 140 mmHg or diastolic > 90 mmHg on 2 occasions at least 4 hours apart in a patient > 20-week gestation
- Previously normotensive[1]
  - Preeclampsia can be superimposed on chronic hypertension

Systolic > 160 mmHg or diastolic > 110 mmHg confirmation within minutes is acceptable AND[1]
- Proteinuria OR new onset hypertension with or without proteinuria if any of the following present[1]:
  - Serum creatinine > 1.1 mg/dL or the creatinine concentration is double without renal disease
  - Thrombocytopenia (platelet count < 100 000/μL)
  - Transaminase liver function tests >twice the upper limit of normal
  - Pulmonary edema
  - Visual or cerebral symptoms (H/A, vision changes)

HELLP syndrome (Hemolysis, Elevated liver enzymes, Low platelets) may be a different disorder or a severe form of preeclampsia

Most new-onset hypertension with proteinuria presents > 34 weeks' gestation[2]
- About 10% are < 34 weeks[2]

■ EVALUATION

May be asymptomatic but exam warning signs include[3]:
- Severe or persistent headache
- Altered mental status
- Vision changes (blurred vision, photophobia)
- Upper abdominal pain
- Dyspnea or retrosternal chest pain
- Rapid weight gain
- Edema
- Hyperreflexia
- Oliguria

Monitor BP

Labs[1]:
- CBC (platelet count)

Chemistries (serum creatinine, electrolytes, uric acid, liver enzymes)
Uric acid is a poor predictor for complications[4]
U/A (protein)
Fetal ultrasound[1]
Fetal growth restriction from depressed uteroplacental perfusion may be present[5]

MANAGEMENT

Admit severe hypertension or severe preeclampsia[1,6]
Consult OB/Gyn
Severe features may require imminent delivery[1,7]
Inpatient monitoring is reasonable for determining candidates for conservative management[8]
Outpatient care is an option for stable preeclampsia without severe elements[9]
Outcomes of outpatient care are limited[10]
Eclampsia occurs in up to 3% with severe preeclamptic signs not managed with antiseizure prophylaxis (magnesium)[11,12]
New onset seizures are a convulsive manifestation of preeclampsia[12,13]

KEY ECLAMPSIA MANAGEMENT

Manage airway—provide oxygen[14]
Position patient on left side
Prevent hypoxia or trauma—pad bedrails
Treat severe hypertension—exact threshold in which emergent treatment should be initiated is unclear[15]
Labetalol 20 mg IV over 2 minutes initial dose
If target not achieved after 10 minutes—40 mg IV over 2 minutes
If target not achieved after 20 minutes—80 mg IV over 2 minutes
May repeat 80 mg IV at 30 minutes & 40 minutes to a maximum of 300 mg
Switch agents if target not achieved
Option instead of repeated dosing:
1–2 mg/min infusion or start after initial 20 mg IV
Hydralazine option: 5 mg IV over 1–2 minutes

Prevent recurrent seizures[16]
- Magnesium sulfate is the drug of choice: 4–6 g IV over 15–20 minutes
  - May give 5 g IM in each buttock (10 g total)[16]
  - After initial load begin 1–2 g/h infusion (max 40 g/24 h)[16]
- Persistent seizures: diazepam 5–10 mg IV q 5–10 min at rate < 5 mg/min to maximum of 30 mg.[17] Eclampsia usually has brief seizures and no focal deficits.

Evaluate for emergent delivery as definitive treatment[1]

Consult OB/Gyn immediately

Consult neurology if no improvement after 10–20 minutes of hypertension & seizure control or if focal neuro deficits occur

Procedural Conscious Sedation 59

□ GENERAL

No absolute indications or contraindications. Mostly utilized when pain or anxiety may be excessive, thus impeding performance

Different levels of sedation (minimal to deep) are routinely performed by emergency providers[1]

Comorbid conditions may increase the risk of adverse events during sedation[2]

- Risk is reduced by using lower dose—dosing at less frequent intervals—slower administration[2,3]

Procedure does not need to be delayed due to fasting[4]

Obtaining informed consent is preferred[4]

Number of clinicians performing the procedure may vary. At a minimum,

- 1 clinician performing the procedure while another medical professional (ie, nurse) monitors the patient status[4]
- Two clinicians for a single procedure remains controversial[4,5]

Most ED physicians do not use a second clinician

■ EVALUATION

Screen for comorbidities & intubation difficulty in case airway control becomes necessary[1]

Prepare consents, equipment, personnel, and medications

■ MANAGEMENT

Establish IV & monitoring equipment

Airway management equipment (bag valve mask—intubation equipment) available including suction & continuous pulse oximetry[5]

Pre-oxygenate with face mask and nasal O_2 is recommended (evidence for benefit is variable)[1]

Pregnant patients—may reduce complications by utilizing:

- Metoclopramide (improves GE sphincter tone reducing gastric volume)
- Pre-procedural hydration
- Oxygenation
- Left lateral recumbent positioning

Hypoventilation is usually brief. May counter using reversal agents, patient stimulation, airway positioning, bag valve mask support, and/or supplemental oxygen

IV Agents:

- Propofol 0.5–1 mg/kg may repeat 0.5 mg/kg every 3–5 minutes[6,7]
  - Sedative—amnestic. No analgesia
  - Onset under 60 seconds—duration 6 minutes
- Ketamine 1–2 mg/kg over 1–2 minutes may repeat 0.25 mg/kg every 3–5 minutes[6]
  - Dissociative sedative—analgesic—amnestic
  - Rapid onset—long half-life—recovery may take 60 minutes
- Etomidate 0.1–0.15 mg/kg may repeat 0.05 mg/kg every 3–5 minutes[8]
  - Sedative—no analgesia
- Midazolam 0.02–0.03 mg/kg over 2–3 minutes (max 2.5 mg initially). Onset 1–2 minutes
  - May repeat after 2–5 minutes[9]
  - If used with fentanyl can cause hypoxia
  - Sedative—anxiolytic. No analgesia
- Fentanyl 0.5–1 mcg/kg may repeat 0.5 mcg/kg every 2 minutes[10]
  - Analgesic. Reduce dose when combining with other agents

Discharge is generally safe 30–40 minutes after the final sedation medication is administered once no adverse effects have occurred[11]

- Most guidelines recommend discharge if the pre-procedure baseline is achieved[11]

GENERAL

Most common source is the lower extremity[1,2]
Risk factors are related to endothelial injury, hypercoagulability, circulatory stasis,[1,2] recent surgery, trauma, immobilization, cancer, obesity, smoker, pregnancy, prior PE, autoimmune disorders
Symptoms range from none to shock. The most common is dyspnea followed by pleuritic pain, cough, and tachycardia[3]

EVALUATION

Establish the likelihood of PE[4,5]
- Calculate the Wells score: scoring guides the necessity for imaging
- Likely (Wells > 4): perform CTA chest
- Unlikely (Wells < or = 4): perform D-dimer
  - D-dimer < 500 ng/mL = PE excluded
  - D-dimer > or = 500 ng/mL = perform CTA chest (V/Q scan optional)

Consider PERC Criteria[6]
- All 8 fulfilled = PE excluded in low probability population of Wells < 2
- All 8 not fulfilled = D-dimer
  - Age < 50 yo
  - HR < 100/min
  - Pulse oximetry > or = 95%
  - No hemoptysis
  - No estrogen use
  - No prior PE or DVT
  - No unilateral leg swelling
  - No trauma/surgery in past 4 weeks

CBC[3]
Chemistries
PT/INR (before anticoagulation)/PTT
ABG if hypoxic (abnormal ABG is common though it is neither sensitive nor specific: hypoxemia has prognostic value)[3]
Consider ECG, BNP, troponin as markers for right ventricular dysfunction, risk stratification, & prognostic indicators
CXR (evaluate other causes—not necessary if doing a CTA)

CTA chest or V/Q scan (see Wells score screening: image if Wells is in the probable category—D-dimer for low-risk rule out)[3]

PE in pregnancy[7,8]

- Pregnant with leg symptoms = Ultrasound LE
  - Positive: treat
  - Negative: CXR
    - Abnormal CXR: CTA
    - Normal CXR: V/Q—**Please note perfusion only V/Q has the lowest radiation vs CT chest**
- Pregnant without leg symptoms = CXR:
  - Abnormal CXR = CTA
  - Normal CXR = V/Q [7]

MANAGEMENT

Treatment options[9]

- Heparin 80 U/kg (or 5000 units) IV then infusion of 18 U/kg/h (or 1000 U/h)[9]
- Enoxaparin 1 to 1.5 mg/kg SQ daily (inpatient)
- Rivaroxaban 15 mg PO BID for 3 weeks (then 20 mg daily)
- Apixaban 10 mg PO BID for 7 days (then 5 mg BID)

Populations requiring specific anticoagulation strategies:

- Malignancy (heparin preferred)
- Pregnancy (adjusted-dose heparin)
- Heparin-induced thrombocytopenia (option: argatroban)
- If coagulation is contraindicated, patient is unstable, patients with IVC filters or patients who fail anticoagulation

GENERAL

Classified by site (cystitis/pyelonephritis) or syndrome (complicated/uncomplicated)[1]

- *E. coli* is the most common cause in 75–95% of the patients[2]

Complicated UTI involves associated factors that increase failure rates such as:

- Males & children
- Underlying metabolic or functional conditions that complicate the course:
  - Urinary obstruction—pregnancy—DM—renal insufficiency—immunosuppression—catheter
  - Hospital-acquired infection—renal transplant

Uncomplicated UTI[2]:

- Afebrile—can tolerate po meds—nonpregnant/premenopausal—no urologic comorbidities or abnormalities
- No flank pain nor suspicion of pyelonephritis

EVALUATION

History[1]:

- Cystitis: dysuria—urgency—frequency—suprapubic pain—hematuria less common
- Pyelonephritis: also may have fever—chills, flank pain, nausea/vomiting[3]

Pelvic exam if vaginitis or PID suspected

Labs[2,4]:

- U/A (with HCG if childbearing age)
  - Analyze for nitrites, leukocyte esterase, & pyuria confirmed by microscopic evaluation
  - Pyuria may be absent if infection does not communicate with collecting system or is obstructed
- Urine culture (especially if there is pyelonephritis or symptoms recur)[4]
- Chemistries (BUN/creatinine) to assess renal function in pyelonephritis[4]

Consider CBC

Imaging generally not required unless there is obstruction, an anatomic abnormality is suspected, or symptoms not improved after 48–72 hours[5,6]

- CT or renal ultrasound is useful with non-contrasted CT becoming standard[5,7]

MANAGEMENT

Consult local antibiogram

Uncomplicated cystitis (not for a complicated course—cultures can guide therapy)[8]:
- Nitrofurantoin 100 mg BID 5 days
- Fosfomycin trometamol 3 g po single dose
- Trimethoprim-sulfamethoxazole (TMP-SMX) DS BID 3 days (acceptable if early pyelonephritis)
- Ciprofloxaxin 500 mg BID
- Levofloxacin 750 mg daily 5–7 days

Uncomplicated pyelonephritis (consider IV dose before transition to po):[9]
- Levofloxacin 750 mg IV or po daily for 5 days
- Ciprofloxacin 400 mg IV or 500 mg po BID for 10 days
- Consider TMP-SMX DS BID for 14 days if susceptible organism
  - Consider cetriaxone 1 g IV before transition to po TMP-SMX DS
- Consider phenazopyridine 200 mg TID for a max 2 days for relief of symptoms

Complicated pyelonephritis (options guided by cultures) include[8]:
- Ceftriaxone 1 g q 24 h IV
- Cefepime 2 g q 12 h IV
- Piperacillin–tazobactam 3.375 g q 6 h IV
- Imipenem 500 mg q 6 h IV

Insufficient evidence cranberry juice treats UTIs[10]

Admit complicated pyelonephritis[11]
- Indications include: complicated infections—sepsis—persistent vomiting—failed outpatient treatment—extremes of age[11]
- Typical in-patient treatment: fluoroquinolone, aminoglycoside, or third-generation cephalosporin[11]
- Mortality lower for in-patient management[12]

GENERAL

Pasteurella is the most common isolate in cats & dogs[1,2]
Streptococcus & *Staphylococcus* species are also common[1,2]
Streptococcus anginosus is the most common isolate in human bite study with 54% having both aerobic & anaerobic isolates[3]
Bartonella henselae is responsible for the cat-scratch disease
Infections due to a single isolate are rare[6]

EVALUATION

Assess Td status
Assess time of injury, penetration to joint, nerve, tendon, or presence of FB
Assess for immunocompromised conditions
Determine if bite was provoked for rabies exposure
Determine human bite exposures: Hepatitis B, Hepatitis C, syphilis, HIV (note: transmission of HIV through saliva is rare)[1,4]
Determine if bite was provoked or not provoked assessing for rabies exposure in dog bites. Assess for clenched-fist injury in human bite. Systemic symptoms of infection may not occur for 24–72 hours[1,4]
An x-ray may identify a fracture or FB
CT for deep dog bites to scalp[5]
Diagnostic value of labs for infected wounds is unclear but usually not performed clinically: CBC, CRP, ESR[4]
Wound culture may be helpful for infected wounds[1,4]

MANAGEMENT

Clean under local anesthesia—copious irrigation
Debridement of devitalized tissue
Closure controversial:
- Simple dog bites & facial lacerations are generally closed if: < 12 hours old (24 hours face), but not on the hand nor foot, and not if infected
- Do not close: cat, human bites (except on face), crush injuries, punctures, hands, feet, immunocompromised[6]

Prophylactic antimicrobials are controversial:
  Recommended for high-risk wounds—moderate to severe, crush, deep punctures, hands, feet, human bites, and immunocompromised[4,7]
Amoxicillin/clavulanic acid (dog, cat, human)
  Alternative if PCN allergic—TMP-SMZ or doxycycline plus metronidazole or clindamycin
Admit systemic illness, clenched-fist injury (may need OR), or severe bites (if less severe may follow-up in 24 hours)[8]
Assess Td & animal potential for rabies
Consider Hep B vaccine & HIV prophylaxis in human bites
Consider rabies Immunoglobulin (RIG) and vaccine if cannot monitor the animal
RIG 20 IU/kg: Infiltrate around wound then remaining IM and
Vaccine 1 mL IM (adult): Days 0, 3, 7, and 14 per CDC Rec (duration of immunity is > 2 years)
Bats are a concerning vector in the US
Small rodents—squirrels, guinea pigs, hamsters, chipmunks, gerbils, rats, & mice including lagomorphs (rabbits) are almost never found to be infected with rabies & have not been known to transmit rabies to humans according to the CDC
In all cases involving rodents, the state or local health dept should be consulted for the latest report before deciding to initiate treatment

Radial Head Subluxation 63

GENERAL

Typically 1–4 yo[1]
  Range reported from 6 months to 11 yo
Pulling arm in extension is the classic mechanism—falls, minor elbow trauma, and play injuries are also reported[1]
Typical history is that of a child not using the affected arm[1]

EVALUATION

Exam: arm held pronated close to body—passive elbow range of motion if permitted by a cooperative child is normal
  Pain on even minimal supination is always present
  Significant swelling, tenderness, or deformity could suggest a supracondylar fracture
  Be sure to examine clavicle to wrist (clavicle fractures can be missed)
X-ray: this is a clinical diagnosis—x-ray is usually not needed if presentation & exam are consistent with the diagnosis[2]
  Classic "pulling" history with slightly flexed elbow & pronated forearm without bony tenderness, deformity, or swelling
  X-ray indicated[1,2]: direct trauma mechanism of injury
    Swelling (except minimal at radial head)
    Focal bony tenderness or deformity
    Inability to reduce a presumed subluxation

MANAGEMENT

Two methods (there is limited evidence that the hyperpronation method may be less painful with a higher success rate with first attempt)[3,4]
  A click may be felt by a finger over the radial head when reduced
  Hyperpronation method: support elbow with moderate pressure on the radial head with a finger. Then hyperpronate the forearm using the other hand. May grasp as if shaking hands. May flex elbow if not initially successful
  Supination method: support elbow with moderate pressure on the radial head with a finger. Then exert gentle forearm traction using the other hand while fully supinating and fully flexing the elbow in one motion

Reduction is successful if the child moves arm about 5–10 minutes after the procedure—though initially they may be reluctant
- Entice the child to reach for the toy with the affected arm

If unwilling to move arm—x-ray if no initial x-rays were obtained
- Treat fracture if noted
- If no fracture—follow-up in a few days to assess arm movement

If reduction successful—no further treatment necessary, although the risk of future subluxation is increased

☐ GENERAL

Standard of care—sequential administration of sedative & paralytic agent—improves success—reduces complications[1]

RSI contraindications are relative, though each drug may have contraindications

■ EVALUATION

Determine the risk of the difficult airway (anatomic features/clinical findings/Mallampati score)

■ MANAGEMENT

Prepare equipment & medications[2]
- Have a backup method prepared for airway control

Pre-oxygenate
- Goal is to tolerate a longer period of apnea
- Cooperative patients taking deep breaths achieves nitrogen washout[3]
- Reserve manual ventilation for hypoxic (< 91% sats) patients
- Extremity pulse ox readings will lag behind central arterial circulation readings[4]

Pretreat with any meds to mitigate adverse effects

Administer induction agents & paralytics

Cricoid pressure to prevent passive regurgitation has questionable effectiveness[5]

Confirm placement after intubation
- End-tidal CO_2 is the most accurate
- Do not rely on a single indicator (cord visualization, auscultation, tube mist)
- CXR can only determine depth. It is not useful to distinguish endotracheal placement

64 Rapid Sequence Intubation

SOAP-ME mnemonic

Suction: good suction available (short tubing)

Oxygen: pretreat-BVM 15 L/min—passive oxygen via nasal cannula (5 L/min) during apneic period extends saturation[1]

Airway: ET tube (8.0 male:7.5 female): good light on handle

Positioning: sniffing position/pre-oxygenation: non-rebreather 4 minutes prior: good bed height: calm demeanor

Monitoring/med: pulse ox, cardiac monitoring

End-tidal CO_2

MEDS

IV Sedation/induction

- Etomidate 0.3–0.4 mg/kg (150 lb = **20 mg**)
  - Not peds approved
- Midazolam 0.1–0.3 mg/kg (150 lb = **6–20 mg**)
  - Post intubation versed drip 4–6 mg/h
- Propofol 1–2.5 mg/kg (150 lb = **70–170 mg**)
- Fentanyl 2–10 mcg/kg (150 lb = **100–600 mcg**)
  - May start 50 mcg—↑ q 3 min to effect: conscious sedation)
  - Post intubation Fentanyl drip 50–100 mcg/h

IV Paralytics

- Succinylcholine 1–2 mg/kg (150 lb = **100 mg**)
  - Malignant hyperthermia can occur in contraindicated patients.
- Rocuronium 0.6–1.2 mg/kg (150 lb = **40–80 mg**)

IV Adjunct agents

- Ketamine 1–4.5 mg/kg (150 lb = **70–300 mg** over 1–2 minutes)
  - Peds = 1.5 mg/kg over 1–2 minutes: (3–4 mg/kg IM: conscious sedation)
- Lidocaine 1.5–2 mg/kg (150 lb = **100–130 mg**)
  - Consider in head injury

GENERAL

Respiratory illness affecting all ages with seasonal outbreaks
  Most children have been infected by 2 yo—reinfection is common[1]
Most common lower respiratory tract infection in children age < 1 yo[2]
  Adult occurrence is significant & is often unrecognized[3]
URI prodrome, wheezing, increased respiratory effort[4]
Direct contact with secretions (nasopharynx/mucus membranes) is the primary mode of transmission, though aerosolized droplets have been noted—can survive several hours on hands and surfaces such as clothes[5]
Apnea can occur in infants by an unknown mechanism[6]
  RSV has been suggested as a possible cause of sudden infant death syndrome[7]

EVALUATION

URI prodrome is several days—rhinitis, cough, fever[4]
  Progression next several days—wheezing or respiratory distress
CBC (WBC) does not predict bacteremia & is not clinically useful in guiding treatment[8,9]
RSV antigen testing[9]
Urine (< 90 days old)[10]
CXR (does not correlate well to the severity of disease—needed if there is significant respiratory effort or a complication is suspected)[4]
  FB aspiration, heart failure, pneumonia
Pulse oximetry

MANAGEMENT

Oxygen if needed (nasal)
  Optional if $SpO_2 > 93\%$
Assess hydration needs
Assess risk factors for poor outcomes
  History of prematurity
  Age < 12 weeks
  Cardiopulmonary disease
  Immunodeficiency

Bronchiolitis that is not severe can typically be managed as an outpatient unless there are social concerns
- Bronchodilators, glucocorticoids, & leukotriene inhibitors have no proven benefit[4,11-13]
- Antimicrobials should not be used unless there is a concomitant bacterial infection[4]
- Supportive care is the recommended treatment: the course is usually 2-3 weeks with a peak of 3-5 days
  - Nasal suctioning
  - Po hydration as intake is generally decreased
  - Avoid OTC decongestants
  - Precautions to return if poor feeding, distress, or worse symptoms

Admit severe cases
- Trial of inhaled bronchodilator (including epinephrine)
- Heated humidified high-flow HFNC & CPAP are beneficial, and reduce intubation rates[14]
  - Intubate if hypoxemic despite O_2, impending respiratory failure or apnea
- Heliox may be beneficial[15]
- Corticosteroids improved clinical scores slightly for inpatients especially with inhaled epinephrine, but not outpatients[16]
- Do not use nebulized hypertonic saline in the ER[4,17]

Typical ER or inpatient discharge criteria:[18]
- Respiratory rate < 60/min age < 6 months—< 55/min age 6–11 months—< 45/min age > 12 months
- Stable without supplement O_2 at least 12 hours before discharge
  - Sats > 92%[19]
- Caregiver can suction nose
- Adequate family support
- Adequate po hydration

☐ GENERAL

Causation: Rickettsia rickettsii, gram-negative. Infected patients become symptomatic 2–14 days after exposure from tick bite as the primary vector Virulence occurs after the tick ingests a blood meal or after 1–2 days

Do not be fooled by the name—it is most common in **North Carolina** and **Oklahoma**

One-third of patients do not recall a bite[1,2]

Increased mortality (22.9% vs 6.5%) if the delay of antimicrobial institution exceeds 5 days

Males, Native Americans, and frequent exposure to dogs or wooded areas are some of the highest reported cases[2]

April–Sept is the peak incidence, but you can get it year round

Children < 10 yo, Native Americans, immunocompromised, & delayed treatment increases the risk of a fatal outcome[2]

Increased mortality if there is a delay of antimicrobial treatment[3]

■ EVALUATION

Clinical manifestations include headache, fever, and rash after tick exposure[4]

Commonly mistaken as viral illness initially

Incubation period: 2–14 days

Children may have GI symptoms such as nausea/vomiting[5]

Most develop a rash between 3–5 days of illness (10% have no rash). Rash typically begins at ankles/wrists and spreads centrally to palms/soles

No reliable early test. Serologic dx should be regarded as retrospective confirmation[6]

CBC not diagnostically helpful. Thrombocytopenia may be more prevalent as the illness progresses

Hyponatremia, increased serum aminotransferases, bilirubin, and prothrombin time prolongation may occur in advanced cases

Antibodies appear 7–10 days after the onset of the illness. The optimal time to obtain convalescent antibody titer is at 14–21 days. Serologic testing is not helpful during the first 5 days when therapy should be initiated[3]

■ MANAGEMENT

RMSF should be considered in febrile patients in endemic areas with known or possible tick bite presenting with **headache & fever**/constitutional symptoms in spring or summer. Waiting for rash is not advisable before initiating an empiric treatment

Treatment: doxycycline 100 mg po BID continued at least 3 days after the patient is afebrile. Most are cured in 5–7 days with antibiotics[3]

Doxycycline also 1st line for children < 8 yo with suspected RMSF[7]

If suspected empiric treatment with doxycycline for RMSF should be initiated in symptomatic patients

Pregnant women may be given chloramphenicol (50 mg/kg/d po in 4 divided doses)[8]

Children—the risk of dental staining is minimal with doxycycline if a short course is administered. The risk must be weighed against fatal aplastic anemia due to chloramphenicol therapy

Children weighing more than 45 kg should receive the adult dose of doxycycline

< 45 kg: 2.2–4 mg/kg/d (up to 200 mg/d) BID (duration: 1 week minimum RMSF 2–3 week Lyme)[9,10]

Observation of mildly ill febrile patients can be justified during the first 3 days of illness

Most treated patients will defervesce within 48–72 hours

Hospitalization is dependent on severity—particularly those with complications, such as hypotension, seizures, or marked GI symptoms. It is difficult to distinguish meningococcal infection and RMSF; therefore, if suspected empiric treatment should be initiated in ill pts[10]

Prophylactic treatment is not indicated for those traveling to endemic areas or those who have had a tick bite but have no symptoms[9]

☐ GENERAL

Use of prescription medication for unintended purposes is misuse
- Diversion is obtaining, sharing, or selling prescription drugs
- Any criminal act involving a prescription drug is a diversion

Obtaining or attempting to obtain controlled substances under false pretenses or misrepresentation is unlawful in many states

Substance use disorder has replaced terms such as substance abuse and dependence
- Heavy use over time is a reasonable definition that reduces stigmatization[1]

Prescription misuse has increased as therapeutic prescribing has increased
- There has now been a decline in opioid prescribing[2]

■ EVALUATION

Risk factors for drug misuse (specifically opioids) include[3,4]:
- History of ETOH or cocaine abuse
- Drug-related convictions, incarceration, or legal problems
- Personal or family history of substance use disorder
- Mental health disorder
- Caucasian

Patients receiving opioid therapy are 4 times more likely to have opioid use disorder than the general population[5]

Controlled substances should be prescribed only if the benefits outweigh risks[6,7]
- Predictive data concerning benefit vs harm is limited

There are no quality trials identifying that opioids are superior to NSAIDs for noncancer or chronic pain[8]
- Selective use of opioids is recommended for acute pain[8]

Determine patient's current usage pattern, recent prescriptions for controlled substances, & availability/access to these prescriptions (any dosage units left)

Attempt third-party confirmation if possible regarding patient's usage pattern to verify patient's access or lack of access to prescriptions that the patient claims to have or not have (many states allow centralized database access)

MANAGEMENT

Identify the cause of pain & institute specific treatment
NSAIDs are first-line agents for acute mild to moderate pain[9]
- Caution is advised when prescribing controlled substances due to the rising misuse & diversion[9]
- Limit to lowest effective dose

Limit dosage units and number of prescriptions when prescribing opiates[10]
- More dosage units & repeat prescriptions (refills) increases the risk of overdose[10]

Many states have controlled substance databases that should be accessed prior to prescribing
- Develop policies to address diversion if the patient seems to be attempting to obtain controlled substances by subterfuge

Drug diversion is a multivictim crime[11]

GENERAL

Aspirin, bismuth subsalicylate, analgesics, oil of wintergreen, and effervescent antacids contain salicylates[1]
Results in platelet dysfunction, nausea & vomiting, hyperventilation, respiratory alkalosis, & eventually metabolic acidosis[2]
Concentrations peak > 4–6 hours in overdose

EVALUATION

Symptoms: tinnitus, N/V, diaphoresis, lethargy, agitation, and in severe cases hyperpyrexia, seizures, & coma[3]
Exam: tachypnea, tachycardia, hyperthermia, confusion, vertigo, diarrhea, vomiting
- Symptoms do not correlate to the level of toxicity[4]

Serum salicylate level
- Fatal toxicity can occur after 10–30 g adult ingestion or 3 g child ingestion[4]
  - Therapeutic range 10–30 mg/dL
  - Intoxication symptoms 40–50 mg/dL
- Measure q 2 h until 2 consecutive levels decrease, falls < 40 mg/dL and asymptomatic

Chemistries
- Creatinine as ASA is renally excreted
- Potassium—if hypokalemia is present, must be treated aggressively as this interferes with alkalinization

CBC (coagulopathy may be present)
Serum lactate (may elevate in severe poisoning)
Monitor for elevated anion gap metabolic acidosis[3]
- Chemistries—ABG—urine pH

Acetaminophen level for evaluation of co-ingestion

MANAGEMENT

Asymptomatic with known ingestion < 125 mg/kg—may discharge[4]
Airway—symptomatic ingestions:
- Avoid intubation unless there is clear respiratory failure (ie, hypoventilation)[5]
- High respiratory rate & minute ventilation are difficult to replicate on a ventilator

- If intubated for hypoventilation ventilator settings should mimic the respiratory rate prior to intubation[5]
- Avoid deep sedation, prolonged neuromuscular blockade, & monitor auto-PEEP[5]

IVF resuscitation unless pulmonary or cerebral edema is present[6]

Activated charcoal (AC) absorbs ASA well[7]

- Given to alert, cooperated patients who can control airway
- Ingestion < 1-hour duration
- Give po AC 1 g/kg (child)
- Give po AC 50 g (adult)

Alkalinization (urine/serum)[8]

- Sodium bicarbonate 1–2 mEq/kg IV
  - Followed by sodium bicarb infusion 100–150 mEq in 1 L of NS with 5% Dextrose (D5W) add 30–40 mEq/L of potassium chloride (KCL) to prevent hypokalemia
  - Titrate to urine pH of 7.5–8
  - Correct or prevent hypokalemia to maintain effectiveness
  - Alkalemia is not a contraindication for sodium bicarbonate treatment

Glucose in altered mental status regardless of serum glucose concentration[9]

- IV dextrose if not able to eat—D50 or add to each liter of fluid to maintain high normal glucose as ASA toxicity may decrease cerebral concentrations[9]

Consider hemodialysis in severe cases (ie, altered mental status, cerebral or pulmonary edema, kidney injury, severe acidemia).[10] Consult nephrology early as well as Poison Control

☐ GENERAL

Systemic reaction to infection that can lead to organ dysfunction[1]

Evolving definitions are not diagnostic, as there are no clear guidelines causally linking the presence of infection to sepsis[2]

Risk factors for septic shock[3]:

- ICU admit (50% have a nosocomial infection)[4]
- Bacteremia (one study had 95% positive blood cultures related to sepsis)[5]
- Age > 65 yo
- Immunosuppression & comorbidities
  - DM—cancer—pneumonia—renal failure
- Previous hospitalization in the last 90 days

A significant percentage of septic patients (289 out of 3563) defined by blood culture had no fever (33%) and a normal WBC (52%)—17% had both no fever & an NL WBC, though bandemia is a useful measure present in 80% of patients with a positive blood cultures[6]

■ EVALUATION

Symptoms are variable and nonspecific[7]

- Fever (or hypothermia), hypotension, tachycardia, leukocytosis, and organ dysfunction such as altered mental status or oliguria (search for infectious sources)

Sequential Organ Failure Assessment (SOFA)[8]

Lungs

PaO_2/FIO_2 > 400	(0 points)
301–400	(1 point)
< 300	(2 points)
101–200 with ventilatory support	(3 points)
< 100 with ventilatory support	(4 points)

Platelets

> 150 × $10^3/mm^3$	0 points
101–150	1 point
51–100	2 points
21–50	3 points
< 20 × 103/mm^3	4 points

Bilirubin

< 1.2 mg/dL (20 mcmol/L)	0 points
1.2–1.9 mg/dL (20–32 mcmol/L)	1 point
2–5.9 mg/dL (33–101 mcmol/L)	2 points
6–11.9 mg/dL (102–204 mcmol/L)	3 points
> 12 mg/dL (> 204 mcmol/L)	4 points

BP

No hypotension	0 points
MAP < 70 mmHg	1 point
On dopamine <= 5 mcg/kg/min or any dobutamine	2 points
On dopamine > 5 mcg/kg/min, epi ≤ 0.1 mcg/kg/min or norepinephrine ≤ 0.1 mcg/kg/min	3 points
On dopamine > 15 mcg/kg/min or epi > 0.1 mcg/kg/min or norepinephrine > 0.1 mcg/kg/min	4 points

Glasgow Coma Score

15	0 points
13–14	1 point
10–12	2 points
6–9	3 points
< 6	4 points

Renal function

Creatinine < 1.2 mg/dL (110 mcmol/L)	0 points
1.2–1.9 mg/dL (110–170 mcmol/L)	1 point
2–3.4 mg/dL (171–299 mcmol/L)	2 points
3.5–4.9 mg/dL (300–440 mcmol/L)	3 points
> 5 mg/dL (440 mcmol) or urine output < 200 mL/d	4 points

Score

0–6	< 10% mortality rate
7–9	15–20%
10–12	40–50%
13–14	50–60%
15	> 80%
15–24	> 90%

The SOFA Score[a]

Organ System, Measurement	SOFA Score				
	0	1	2	3	4
Respiration PaO_2/FiO_2, mm Hg	Normal	< 400	< 300	< 200 (with respiratory support)	< 100 (with respiratory support)
Coagulation Platelets $\times 10^3/mm^3$	Normal	< 150	< 100	< 50	< 20
Liver Bilirubin, mg/dL (µmoL/l)	Normal	1.2–1.9 (20–32)	2.0–5.9 (33–101)	6.0–11.9 (102–204)	> 12.0 (< 204)
Cardiovascular Hypotension	Normal	MAP < 70 mm Hg	Dopamine < 5 or dobutamine (any dose)[b]	Dopamine > 5 or epinephrine < 0.1 or norepinephrine < 0.1	Dopamine > 15 or epinephrine > 0.1 or norepinephrine > 0.1
Central Nervous System Glasgow Coma Score	Normal	13–14	10–12	6–9	< 6
Renal Creatinine, mg/dL (µmoL/l) or urine output	Normal	1.2–1.9 (110–170)	2.0–3.4 (171–299)	3.5–4.9 (300–440) or < 500 mL/d	> 5.0 (> 440) or < 200 mL/d

[a]

[b] Adrenergic agents administered for at least 1 hour (doses given are in mcg/kg/min).

Source: Vincent JL, Moreno R, Takala J, et al. The SOFA (Sepsis-related Organ Failure Assessment) score to describe organ dysfunction/failure. On behalf of the working group on sepsis-related problems of the European Society of Intensive Care Medicine. *Intensive Care Med*. July 1996;22(7):707–710.

CBC—CMP—serial serum lactate—ABG (in hypoxia)—Coag studies—amylase/lipase—U/A & culture—sputum culture (cough)—blood cultures (2 sets), obtain cultures both peripherally & from any indwelling lines—procalcitonin & CRP[9]
Imaging site specific to identify suspected infection (eg, CXR for suspected pneumonia)
SOFA Score

MANAGEMENT

Assess & treat septic shock if present
- Correct hypoxemia—establish IV access (fluids/antimicrobials)

Initiate fluid resuscitation > 30 mL/kg within 1st 3 hours (2 L for 150 lbs adult)[9]
- Evidence of pulmonary edema may be exception to rapid fluid infusion

Begin broad-spectrum antibiotics or guided by a source within the 1st hour
- Piperacillin-tazobactam
- Carbapenem
- Vancomycin (MRSA suspected)[10]

Consider combination therapy from 2 different drug classes
Consider vasopressors (norepinephrine/Levophed)[11]
- Dopamine may be used with low risk of tachyarrhythmia
- Vasopressin a choice for less severe sepsis

Consider dobutamine (up to 20 mcg/kg/min) if myocardial dysfunction or persistent hypoperfusion[12]
- Can be used while using other vasopressors
- Also appropriate for those not in septic shock (low cardiac output but preserved MAP)

Place central line as soon as feasible or indicated
RBC infusion if Hgb < 7
- Earlier transfusion may be necessary for signs of tissue hypoperfusion, severe hypoxemia, myocardial infarction, or ischemic heart disease[7]

Source control measures (remove infected caths, I/D abscesses)
Corticosteroids suggested (200 mg/d) only when hypotension responds poorly to fluids & vasopressors[9]

70 Sore Throat

☐ GENERAL

Group A Strep (GAS) is the primary etiology
- Rarer treatable causes: gonococcal, H. influenza type B, diptheria[1]
- Vaccinations have decreased diptheria cases in the US. In the past decade < 5 cases reported in the US[2]
- Epstein–Barr virus (EBV) is a notable nonbacterial origin causing mononucleosis[3]

Treatment goals: decreases symptoms if begun < 2 days of illness, reduces complications (abscesses), reduces incidence of rheumatic fever, glomerulonephritis, & close contact transmission

■ EVALUATION

Centor score for adults (modify +1 if < 15 yo: −1 if > 45 yo)[4,5]
1. History of fever
2. Tonsillar exudate
3. Tender anterior cervical lymphadenopathy
4. Absence of cough

All criteria = empiric treatment (note: PCN is cheaper than test)
3 criteria = empiric tx or rapid antigen test with tx only if positive
2 criteria = rapid antigen test—Tx only if positive—*or* no test—no tx
1 criteria = no test—no tx

Suggestive Findings

Palatine petechiae or scarlatiniform rash:	Consider Strep
Strep exposure past 2 weeks or duration < 3 days:	Consider Strep
Headache, stiff neck, petechial rash:	Consider meningitis
Hot-Potato voice, sudden severe sx, trismus:	Consider peritonsilar abscess
Posterior cervical lymphadenopathy or teenager:	Consider mononucleosis
"Woody" submandibular induration:	Consider Ludwig's angina
Red swollen uvula (can be associated with GAS):	Consider uvulitis

MANAGEMENT

Pen VK 250 mg po QID or 500 mg BID for 10 days for adults
  250 mg BID or TID for children
Benzathine Pen G 1.2 million units IM once (600 000 if wt < 27 kg/60 lbs)
Amoxil 50 mg/kg/d po (max 1000 mg) or 25 mg/kg (max 500 mg) BID × 10 days
If PCN allergic:
  Cephalexin 20 mg/kg po BID (max 500 mg)
  Clindamycin 7 mg/kg po TID (max 300 mg): also used for recurrent GAS[6]
  Azithromycin 12 mg/kg po once daily (max 500 mg) for 5 days
  Erythromycin 40 mg/kg/po day in 2–4 doses (400 mg QID adults)
NSAIDs/acetaminophen
Dexamethasone 0.6 mg/kg IV/IM (max 10 mg) once for symptom relief
  Not recommended by Infectious Disease Society
  However, it has been studied favorably in the Emergency Medicine Literature including the Cochrane Review[7–10]
Informing patients that they will feel better after 24 hours increases the subjective cure rate[11]
Rinsing or changing toothbrush may reduce failure rates[12]
Prophylaxis is not routinely recommended for family members unless there is a history of rheumatic fever[13,14]

71 Superficial Thrombophlebitis

☐ GENERAL

Thrombosis & inflammation of a superficial vein that is warm, painful, erythematous, and tender with a palpable cord usually in lower extremities but can occur anywhere. Significant portion also has DVT, PE, or may develop further complications

Suspect superficial vein thrombosis (SVT) tender when there is inflammation along the superficial vein, varicose veins, recent trauma, immobilization, pregnancy, malignancy, or a hypercoagulable state. Consider the potential for DVT or PE

Commonly of the LE. May occur at site of IV

Risk factors: varicose veins, elderly > 60 yo, immobilization, obese, pregnancy, IV infusion, endothelial dysfunction, cancer, history of thrombosis or thrombophilia[1]

Duplex ultrasound enables the distinction between phlebitis and thrombophlebitis by differentiating the presence of a clot

Risk of MI, CVA, and death may increase following SVT diagnosis

- Whether SVT of lower extremity increases thrombotic events such as DVT or PE risk is uncertain[2]

■ EVALUATION

Ultrasound to confirm SVT & assess for DVT[3]

- Perform if study will change management[4]
- Saphenous vein involvement requires ultrasound[5,6]
- DVT can be present in conjunction with SVT
  - SVT close to the deep vein system has a high prevalence of concomitant proximal DVT[7]

Uncomplicated phlebitis not affecting the saphenous vein area with no other DVT risk factors may not require ultrasound[5,6]

Perform US if phlebitis occurs in the lower extremity with a central catheter (groin) evaluating for DVT[7]

D-dimer has low sensitivity for SVT as thrombotic burden felt to be less than DVT

CBC, blood cultures for suppurative phlebitis

Screening for hypercoagulability in a single episode is not cost effective due to the low yield, but is a consideration in recurrent episodes specifically for the patients undergoing malignancy evaluation[8]

MANAGEMENT

Treatment is symptomatic & prevention of venous thromboembolism (SVT increases thromboembolism risk)[9]

Uncomplicated (thrombus < 5 cm, remote from saphenous vein, no medical risk factors) requires symptomatic treatment & support[10,11]
- Elevate LE: compression/support stockings
- Compresses (warm or cool): remain ambulatory and NSAIDS
- Antimicrobial not indicated unless infected

Treat DVT if present

If DVT is not present but thrombus is within 3 cm of saphenous-femoral junction or if thrombus > 5 cm—consider as equivalent to DVT[10–12]

Systemic anticoagulation for 45 days if[10–12]:
- SVT of the lower limb is > 5 cm in length, recommendation is prophylactic dose of fondaparinux or LMWH for 45 days over no anticoagulation
- SVT within 3 cm of sapheno-femoral junction should be considered for anticoagulation

Anticoagulation is not typically used to treat IV infusion associated SVT[13,14]

There are no RCTs to direct management of upper extremity superficial thrombosis[13–15]

72 Syncope

☐ GENERAL

Majority of cases have an unknown etiology[1]
Cardiac & unknown etiology increases the risk of death. Vasovagal syncope typically has a benign prognosis[1]
Defined as the self-terminating inadequacy of global cerebral nutrient perfusion (transient loss of consciousness [TLOC])[2]

Broad categories	Neural-mediated (vasovagal)
	Orthostatic (autonomic)
	Cardiac (arrhythmia)

Syncope should be distinguished from other TLOC causes due to its pathophysiology
Other TLOC conditions include: seizures, intoxication, and concussion
History, physical, & ECG are core evaluations[3]
Neurologic testing rarely adds value unless neurologic symptoms are present[3]
Suspected heart disease or exertional syncope are high-risk factors and need a cardiac workup[3]
Syncope in the elderly is frequently from polypharmacy or physiologic[3]
Micturition and defecation are common etiologies in the elderly
Admission is indicated for suspicion of a cardiac etiology (abnormal ECG, heart disease, CP, arrhythmia, age > 70 yo) or neurologic symptoms[3]

■ EVALUATION

Determine if it is true syncope and the possible etiologies through a detailed history & physical exam[4] and ECG as the core evaluation[4]
If etiology is determined—consider treatment for the etiology & risk assessment.
If it is an unknown etiology—consider further evaluation & risk assessment
Routine testing has low yield unless suspicion exists of contributory conditions[4,5]
ECG, QT interval monitoring, & orthostatic vitals are minimal tests[5]
Neural mediated (orthostatic) requires no further workup[4,5]
Additional testing should be targeted depending on the suspicion of the etiology[4,5]

CBC
Chemistries, accucheck as well
Cardiac panel
HCG in females
Holter monitor may be helpful for frequent episodes
Echocardiography if structural disease is suspected[4]
Neurologic testing (CT & MRI) not recommended in the absence of head injury or neurologic findings[4,6]
Tilt testing may be helpful if positional or reflex etiology is suspected[7]
San Francisco Syncope Rule (CHESS 5 RF). High sensitivity of serious 7-day outcome (1 or more = admission)[8]
History of congestive heart failure
Hematocrit < 30%
Abnormal ECG (any ectopic focus or new changes)
SOB
Systolic BP < 90 mmHg

Diagnostic Predictive Score[9]

Palpitations preceding syncope	+4
Heart disease, abnormal ECG, or both	+3
Syncope during exertion	+3
Precipitating factors (fear, pain, emotion, orthostasis)	−1
Autonomic prodromes (N/V)	−1

Risk of cardiac causes

< 3 points=	2%
3 points=	13%
4 points=	33%
> 4 points=	77%

72 Syncope

MANAGEMENT

Differential Considerations

Cardiac—dysrhythmia, valvular heart disease, aortic dissection, IHSS, steal syndrome, carotid stenosis, vertebrobasilar insufficiency

Neurocardiogenic—cough, defecation, micturition, carotid sinus sensitivity

Neurologic—seizure, TIA/CVA, migraine

Orthostatic—hypovolemia, GI bleed, ectopic pregnancy, heat

Other—hypoglycemia, hypoxia, anemia, psychogenic

Admit: high-risk features—any suspicious serious underlying etiology or unclear etiology of intermediate risk[4]

Consider advancing age, cardiac history, & San Francisco rules[4]

Specifically admit older than 60 yo

Vasovagal (nausea/vomiting, defecation, micturition, positional, pain, psychogenic) if < 60 yo may D/C home[4]

Testicular Torsion 73

GENERAL

Can occur at any age. The most common age is 12–18 yo and is a urological emergency[1,2]
- Torsion is less common than epididymitis, which is the most common etiology of scrotal pain[3]

Abrupt onset of severe pain and N/V have positive predictive value[4]

Scrotum may be edematous, erythematous, tender with a high-riding testicle, and absent cremasteric reflex[5]
- Intermittent torsion can cause intervals during which there is no pain

Salvage rates to detorsion[6]:
- Typically, a 4–8-hour window before permanent ischemia occurs
  - < 6 hours 90–100% salvage rate
  - < 12 hours 50% salvage rate
  - > 24 hours < 10% salvage rate

EVALUATION

Color Doppler ultrasound if torsion suspected[7]

Exclude other causes: epididymitis, orchitis, Fournier's gangrene[6]

Urinalysis (often normal in torsion)[8]

Cremasteric reflex is absent in torsion[5]
- Scrotum elevation may relieve epididymitis pain
- Scrotum elevation may aggravate or have no effect on torsion pain

MANAGEMENT

Consult urology for immediate surgery[6]

Manual detorsion reserved in extenuating circumstances if care > 2 hours away[9,10]
- Open book is the classic technique, though one-third rotate laterally[10]

Torsion of the appendix of the testis (blue dot sign)[11]
- Analgesics, bed rest, scrotal support = resolves in 5–10 days

Epididymitis[12]
- Ceftriaxone 250 mg IM & doxcycline 100 mg po bid × 10 days for age < 35 yo with STD risk, analgesics, bedrest, scrotal elevation/support
- Levofloxacin 500 mg po bid × 10 days for age > 35 yo with low STD risk

Note: Consult urology even with a negative ultrasound due to the possibility of intermittent torsion

74 Threatened Abortion

GENERAL

Presence of vaginal bleeding does not predict spontaneous abortion as bleeding is common in the 1st trimester (20–40%)[1]
- Abortion is the most common complication of early pregnancy

Passage of fetal tissue is generally accompanied by cramping
- Clots can be mistaken for a tissue

EVALUATION

Determine last menstrual period (LMP) to determine gestational age

Pelvic exam to confirm source of bleeding, volume, products of conception, & assess for cervical dilatation

Pelvic ultrasound is the primary diagnostic tool (helps exclude ectopic pregnancy as well)
- Fetal cardiac activity may be detected at 5.5 to 6 weeks[2]

Labs:
- Serum HCG
- Blood type & Rh
  - Rh negative patients with bleeding including spotting should be provided anti-D immunoglobulin (300 mcg IM)[3]
- CBC if significant blood loss

Inevitable abortion: dilated cervix with visualization of products of conception (POC) at the internal os

Incomplete abortion: dilated cervix with visualization of POC within canal

Missed abortion: spontaneous abortion with a closed cervix

MANAGEMENT

Inevitable, incomplete, & missed abortion can be managed surgically or with medical evacuation

No specific management is available to sustain pregnancy in threatened abortion[4]
- Bedrest is advised but there is no evidence to support value

Ensure no other sources of bleeding are present including ectopic

Follow serial HCG testing (48 hours) & US within 1 week[4]
- Serum HCG level is detectable around 11 days after conception (12–14 days urine)
- HCG levels generally double every 48–72 hours then decline & plateau at 8–11 weeks

GENERAL

Thyrotoxicosis is rare & life threatening[1]

- High fever (> 104°F), tachycardia, agitation or confusion, diaphoresis, nausea, vomiting, dyspnea
- Exaggerated hyperthyroidism symptoms

Typically precipitated by an event: infection, childbirth, trauma, drugs, surgery

EVALUATION

Diagnosis: severe symptoms (fever, tachycardia, altered mentation) with evidence of hyperthyroidism

- Usually in women. It can present with atypical chest pain and various arrhythmias
- Elevated free T4 and/or T3 with suppression of TSH
- No universal criteria (Burch & Wartofsky introduced one score criteria in 1993)[2]

TSH

- If TSH below normal—measure T3 & T4

Other tests aimed at determining underlying causes

MANAGEMENT

ICU admission

- Mortality rates range up to 25%[3]

Treatment approaches based on case studies[4]

- IVFs for volume resuscitation
- Propylthiouracil (PTU) 500–1000 mg load po or IV, then 250 mg q 4 h
  - Give iodine at least 1 hour after first antithyroid drug dose to block the thyroid hormone release
    - Potassium iodide 5 gtts q 6 h or Lugol's solution 10 gtts PO
  - May consider lithium 300 mg po if iodine contraindicated
  - PTU is preferred, though methimazole 20 mg po is an option. Both PTU and methimazole decrease thyroid hormone production centrally, but PTU inhibits the peripheral conversion of T4 to T3 as well. However, methimazole has a longer duration of action

Propranolol 60–80 mg po q 4 h (consider 0.5–1 mg slow IV, then 1–2 mg IV q 15 min titrate to heart rate)
Dexamethasone 2 mg IV or hydrocortisone 300 mg IV load, then 100 mg IV q 8 h
Cholestyramine 4 g po qid may prevent thyroid hormone recycling
Consider diuretics if CHF occurs
Acetaminophen for fever—avoid salicylates, which may increase hormone levels

☐ GENERAL

Clinical presentation ranges from no symptoms to critically ill depending on the ingested substance
- Occult ingestion should be considered in unexplained presentations of severe illness[1]

Ages 1–4 yo or history of previous ingestion is the highest risk group[2]

Age < 6 yo account for 81% of ED drug overdose visits[3]
- Fatalities are most often from analgesics and antihistamines, then sedative—hypnotic—antipsychotic meds[3]

■ EVALUATION

Stabilize the patient[4]

Attempt to identify the ingested substance, amount, & timing[4]
- Age 1.5–4.5 yo: "Mouthful" volume = 9.3 mL (range 3.5–29 mL)[5]
- Young children typically ingest single agent[5]

Pulse oximeter

Accu-check

Carboxyhemoglobin level if carbon monoxide (CO) poisoning is suspected
- Pulse oximeter is not an accurate reflection in CO poisonings

Labs
- Rapid accu-check
- ABG if necessary
- Chem 7 and liver panel
- Acetominophen/salicylate levels
- U/A (rhabdomyolysis with myoglobinuria)
  - Urine is also helpful in ethylene glycol ingestion: Ca^{++} oxalate crystals may be seen but not always
  - Ethylene glycol (antifreeze) may reveal fluorescence under woods lamp exam of urine[6]
- ECG
- Toxicology screens
- HCG if strike female of childbearing age
- Radiologic imaging for inhalation exposures (CXR for inhalation/abd ominal series for radiopaque ingestions)

CT has little utility in the evaluation of poisoning, but CT head may be useful for complications such as IC hemorrhage or cerebral edema/injuries

Chocolate-colored blood suggests methemoglobinemia caused by many agents—ask about anesthetics/lidocaine or nitrates, etc[7]

It is not unreasonable to preserve samples of blood, urine, vomitus, & gastric contents for additional analysis[8]

MANAGEMENT

Consult a Poison Control Center

Stabilize & provide supportive care[4]

- Decontamination—antidote therapy directed by causative agent & elimination enhancement[9]
- Supportive care, prevention of absorption, & antidote administration/ elimination facilitation as appropriate[4]

Protect airway

Hypoxemia & hypoglycemia are common causes of altered mental status in overdose[10]

- Empirical administration of hypertonic dextrose solutions (D10, D5NS) & thiamine is favored[10]
- Naloxone reserved for evidence of opioid ingestion[10]
- Flumazenil is best for reversal of therapeutic conscious sedation and select benzodiazepine ingestions—may cause seizures in certain patients who have been on benzodiazepines for a longer period of time[10]

IVF for hypotension management

- Vasopressors if needed[11]

Agitated patients with hypertension can be managed with benzodiazepines[12]

- Use of β-blockers alone not recommended in cocaine toxicity—use benzodiazepines[12]
- Haloperidol supplementation may be necessary[13]

Seizures initially treated with benzodiazepines[14]

- Barbiturates is a second-line treatment[14]
- Phenytoin is not indicated in most poisonings except by agents stabilizing neuronal membranes (propranolol)[14]
  - Phenytoin is potentially harmful in theophylline overdose[14]

Decontamination
- There is no evidence that activated charcoal improves clinical outcomes[15]
- Activated charcoal only in patients with protected airway & typically < 1 hour since ingestion[15]
  - Age up to 1 yo: 10–25 g or 0.5–1 g/kg
  - Age 1–2 yo: 25–50 g or 0.5–1 g/kg (max 50 g)
  - Adults: 25–100 g (50 g usual adult dose)
- Sorbitol is not recommended for children
- Gastric lavage is not recommended unless directed by Poison Control[16]

Antidotes if warranted for specific ingestions[17]

Enhanced elimination if warranted for specific ingestions
- Few studies have examined if enhanced elimination improves outcomes
- Multidose activated charcoal—urine alkalinization—dialysis—hemofiltration—exchange transfusion

Thiamine to prevent Wernicke's encephalopathy[18]

Dextrose (25 g for adults) for hypoglycemia[18]

Naloxone for opioid overdose[18]

Disposition[19]
- Observation (typically 6 hours) until asymptomatic is adequate for only mild toxicity
- All intentional ingestions require psychiatric evaluation
- Consider caregivers ability to monitor at home or potential for neglect[19]
- Admit serious ingestions or ingestions with delayed effects
  - Examples: acetaminophen, mushrooms, toxic alcohols, sustained release drugs, po hypoglycemics, warfarin, and fluoride)

Presence of any 8 criteria predicts complicated course best managed in ICU[20]:
- $PaCO_2 > 45$ mmHg
- Intubation
- Post-ingestion seizures
- Non-sinus cardiac rhythm
- Second- or third-degree AV block
- Systolic BP < 80 mmHg
- QRS duration ≥ 0.12 seconds

Increased risks of death following ingestion[21]
- Respiratory depression—hypotension—arrhythmia—age > 61 yo—abnormal core body temperature—suicide attempt—unresponsive to verbal stimuli

77 Upper Respiratory Infection

☐ GENERAL

The symptoms are largely from an immune response
- Conditions that mimic URI: allergic rhinitis, pharyngitis, influenza, sinusitis, and pertussis

Rhinorrhea, sneezing, nasal obstruction, postnasal drip, throat clearing, sore throat, & cough—caused by a virus
- It is the most frequent illness in western world[1]

Self-limited duration up to 10 days or more—cough may last several weeks[2]

Antibiotics are only for strep pharyngitis or rhinosinusitis[2]

Rhinosinusitis: persistent symptoms > 10 days, severe symptoms, fever, purulent nasal discharge, or facial pain > 3 days or worsening symptoms after the viral illness was improving[2]

No testing or antibiotic needed for bronchitis unless pneumonia is suspected[2]

Sputum color (in patients with cough & no lung disease) does not imply therapeutic guidance[3]

The color of nasal discharge is a weak predictor of viral versus bacterial etiology[4]

■ EVALUATION

Physical exam: rhinorrhea, cough, nasal congestion, sore throat, and low-grade fever[2]
- Average duration 7 days
- Peaks 3–4 days
- May last > 3 weeks

Symptoms suggesting serious illness: difficulty in swallowing, headache, neck stiffness, sore throat > 5 days[5]

Symptoms suggesting nonbacterial rhinitis: nasal congestion, postnasal drip, seasonal trigger, watery rhinorrhea, sneezing, and pruritus of the eyes & nose[5]

Symptoms suggesting bacterial sinusitis: URI symptoms > 10 days, facial pain, fever, and purulent discharge[5]

Inquire regarding immunosuppression risk or recent antibiotic exposure
- Comorbid conditions, age > 65 yo history of rheumatic fever, recent treatment failure, tobacco use, and pregnancy could complicate the course[5]

Radiologic studies are not routinely indicated
- Chest x-ray only if lower respiratory pathology suspected
- Sinus radiographs are not routinely indicated[6]

MANAGEMENT

Follow-up if symptoms progress or change
- Acute otitis media is common in children following URI[7]
- Asthma may be triggered by URI

In general, antibiotics are not indicated for bronchitis nor sinusitis
Acetaminophen for fever
NSAIDs may reduce pain
Nonprescription antihistamines, decongestants may improve symptoms in patients age > 6 yo
- Avoid OTC cold preparations in children age < 6 yo[8]

Humidified air not well studied but may benefit[9]
Intranasal steroids have not been found to be effective at relieving URI symptoms[10]

78 Urinary Retention

☐ GENERAL

Etiologies—obstructive, infectious/inflammatory, pharmacologic, & neurologic
- Incidence increases with age (men in their 70s have 10% chance—in their 80s have 30% chance)[1]
- Most common obstructive cause: BPH 53% (other obstructive causes 23%)[2]
- Most common infectious cause: acute prostatitis (Gram neg: *E. coli*, proteus)[3]

■ EVALUATION

Bladder scan/ultrasound with catheterization[1] (scan has high agreement with cath)[4]

Cath is both diagnostic & therapeutic (should be placed if symptomatic)

Ultrasound finding of post-void residual urine considered significant, it varies in the literature from 50–300 mL[1,5]

It is reasonable to use a catheter if exam is strongly suggestive. Ultrasound if the diagnosis is less clear

Bladder vol > 300–400 mL in a patient unable to void suggests retention, but subjective complaints/patient's history is more important as accuracy of ultrasound varies with body habitus (bladder may be palpable with > 200 mL)

Rectal exam for evaluation of BPH & fecal impaction

Labs: Evaluation of renal function/urine: electrolytes (BUN/creatinine), U/A with culture[1]

PSA is not helpful in the acute setting[1]

CT abdominal/pelvis for suspected pelvic mass or malignancy[1]

CT head for suspected intracranial lesion (MRI preferred in multiple sclerosis)[1]

MRI spine for suspected cauda equina, spinal abscess, and spinal cord compression[1]

■ MANAGEMENT

Catheter for relief & volume assessment
- Volume > 300–400 mL in 15 minutes typically leave in
- Volume 200–400 mL may leave in depending on clinical presentation
- Volume < 200 mL urinary retention less likely—other causes for discomfort should be explored

Immediate removal with voiding trial is appropriate for volume < 200 mL

Rapid & complete decompression is adequate as studies show that partial relief with clamping does not reduce complications & actually may increase the risk of UTI[6]

There are no consistent guidelines for suprapubic bladder decompression if initial urethral catheterization is unsuccessful

Urethral catheterizaion is contraindicated in patients with recent urologic surgery—suprapubic catheter is generally placed by a urologist

Empiric antimicrobial treatment is not indicated for an indwelling cath[7]

Consider 5-α-reductase inhibitor (finasteride 5 mg) **and** an α-blocker (tamsulosin 10 mg) for presumed BPH

Rationale for both—the prostate is 50% muscular and 50% glandular

Tamulosin affects the muscle—works very quickly. Finasteride affects the gland—works slowly—takes 6 months for peak effect[8–10]

F/U with urology in 7–10 days

Duration of catheter placement studies have contradictory findings with best success at ~7 days[11]

Diagnoses that warrant probable admission include sepsis, malignancy obstruction, myelopathy, or acute renal failure[12]

VENTILATOR SETTINGS

☐ GENERAL

CPAP (continuous positive airway pressure)
- Increases oxygenation & decreases work of breathing
- Increases intrathoracic pressure decreasing preload and cardiac workload
- Useful in CHF & sleep apnea
- No ventilatory support

BiPAP (bilevel positive airway pressure)
- Pressure differences: inspiratory & expiratory
- Provides ventilatory support
- Useful in COPD exacerbation, HF, and pneumonia

The trial of BiPAP is reasonable if emergent intubation is not required & the problem typically responds to BiPAP[1,2]

BiPAP is often underutilized especially in cases of pulmonary edema & hypercapnia
- pH < 7.30
- $PaCO_2$ > 45 mmHg
- Pulmonary edema from cardiac etiology
- Hypoxemia due to respiratory failure
- COPD exacerbation with hypercapnia

■ EVALUATION

The need for emergent intubation is an absolute contraindication

Contraindications[3]:
- Cardiac arrest
- Pt cannot protect airway
- Life-threatening organ failure (non-respiratory)
- Severe impairment of consciousness
- High risk of aspiration
- Facial deformity
- Anticipating prolonged ventilation
- Recent esophageal anastomosis

■ MANAGEMENT

Begin with low BiPAP settings—gradually increase to relieve symptoms—supplement with oxygen to maintain sats > 90%

- Respiratory therapy to titrate
- Set FiO_2 21–50% to desired SaO_2 (88% typical for known PCO_2 retainers: > 90% for all others)

Inspiratory pressure 8–12 cm H_2O (eg, start IPAP @10) max 20

Expiratory pressure 3–5 cm H_2O (eg, start EPAP @4) max 10

If blowing off CO_2 will need a wider gap between IPAP & EPAP, it usually should not exceed 20 to prevent esophageal blockage

Mechanical ventilator guidelines:

- Trigger: −1 mmHg (will deliver full breath with little effort)
- Resp rate: initial 18
- Tidal volume: typical max 6–8 mL/kg (70 kg = 420–560 tidal volume) > 10 mL/kg risk of barotrauma
- PEEP: start 5 mmHg (if high intercranial pressure concern: keep PEEP low)
- Flow rate: 60 L/min typical, flow rate higher if trying to blow off CO_2 devoting more to expiration
- Inspired O_2 fraction to maintain: sats > 90% and PaO_2 > 60
  - Start typically 100% FiO_2

For patients with asthma ask respiratory to place the patient on a square wave form to allow him or her to have as much time to expire as possible

Each 1 L/min increase in O_2 flow rate increases FiO_2 4%

O_2 flow, L/min	FiO_2, %
1	24
2	28
3	32
4	36
5	40
6	44
7	48
8	52
9	56
10	60

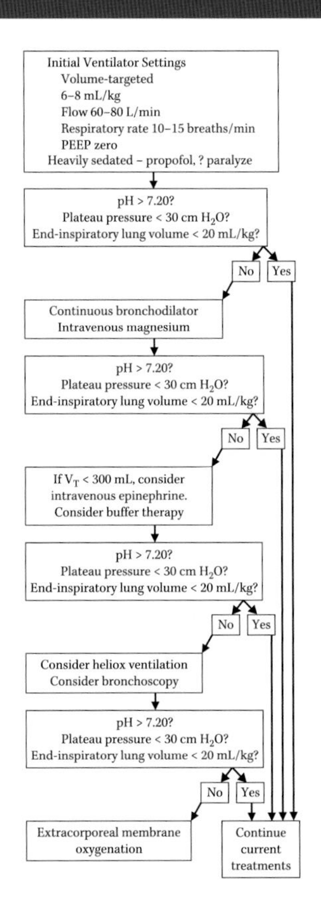
Initial Ventilator Settings
Volume-targeted
6–8 mL/kg
Flow 60–80 L/min
Respiratory rate 10–15 breaths/min
PEEP zero
Heavily sedated – propofol, ? paralyze
pH > 7.20?
Plateau pressure < 30 cm H_2O?
End-inspiratory lung volume < 20 mL/kg?
No
Yes
Continuous bronchodilator
Intravenous magnesium
pH > 7.20?
Plateau pressure < 30 cm H_2O?
End-inspiratory lung volume < 20 mL/kg?
No
Yes
If V_T < 300 mL, consider intravenous epinephrine.
Consider buffer therapy
pH > 7.20?
Plateau pressure < 30 cm H_2O?
End-inspiratory lung volume < 20 mL/kg?
No
Yes
Consider heliox ventilation
Consider bronchoscopy
pH > 7.20?
Plateau pressure < 30 cm H_2O?
End-inspiratory lung volume < 20 mL/kg?
No
Yes
Extracorporeal membrane oxygenation
Continue current treatments

☐ GENERAL

Seek etiology—especially life-threatening conditions: bowel obstruction, pancreatitis, mesenteric ischemia, and MI[1]
Understand complications (fluid depletion, hypokalemia, and alkalosis)[1]
Target therapy (such as relieve underlying cause) or treat symptoms[1]
Viral gastroenteritis is a common cause

■ EVALUATION

Significant clinical features[2]

- Abdominal pain suggests organic etiology—such as, cholecystitis
- Vomiting food hours later suggests gastric outlet obstruction or gastroparesis
- Distention & tenderness along with vomiting suggest bowel obstruction
- Heartburn with nausea suggests GERD[3]
- Early morning vomiting is characteristic of pregnancy[4]
- Vertigo & nystagmus suggests vertiginous etiology—that is, vestibular neuritis, and BPV
- Feculent vomiting suggests obstruction or fistula
- Vomiting with headache may be associated with migraine, or a brain tumor
- Neurogenic origin may be projectile and have neurologic symptoms
- Bulimic vomiting is associated with dental erosion[5]
- Multiple persons that are closely associated and have similar vomiting may indicate the same source

Focus diagnostic tests based on history[6,7]
Also see Chapter 2 (Abdominal Pain)
CBC: identify infection, hydration, anemia
Chemistries: identify hydration, electrolyte imbalance
Urine HCG: pregnancy in females
Drug Levels: toxicity of medications/drug screens
Lipase: pancreatic enzyme levels

Many cases (especially children with gastroenteritis) do not require laboratory investigation[8]
Supine & upright KUB if obstruction is suspected[6]
CT abdomen/pelvis is an option for high suspicion of obstruction or mass
Ultrasound is useful for suspected cholelithiasis or renal pathology
MRI for unexplained chronic vomiting for intracranial mass[6]

■ MANAGEMENT

Rehydration—po or IV depending on clinical presentation[6]
- Estimated 24-hour fluid maintenance needs = 1500 mL plus 20 mL/kg for each kg > 20 kg[6]
- Avoid fluid overload in cardiac patients
- Avoid rapid correction of hyponatremia

Improvement of symptoms & treatment satisfaction similar with ondansetron, metoclopramide, & placebo[8]

Treat underlying cause

Meds

Zofran ($5HT_3$ receptor antagonist) 4 mg IV/PO
- Safety in pregnancy questionable[9,10]

Phenergan (promethazine) 12.5–25 mg IV (sedation caution)
- Irritating to veins. Not recommended for first line[11]

Compazine (phenothiazine) 5–10 mg IV

Reglan (dopamine receptor antagonist: antiemetic & prokinetic) 10 mg IV over 15 minutes to decrease the risk of extrapyramidal effects

Isopropyl alcohol vapor inhalation[12]

Antiemetics may be ineffective in chronic functional nausea: consider antidepressants[13]

☐ GENERAL

There is sufficient evidence in young children exposed to anticoagulant rodenticides to conclude that routine INR measurement is not necessary and should be measured 36–48 hours postexposure (contact Poison Control Center)[1-3]
- Children metabolize warfarin more rapidly than adults with INR quickly returning to normal[3]
- Typical rodenticide treatment plan (contact Poison Control Center):
- INR < 4 & no active bleeding: no action
- Active bleeding: prothrombin complex concentrate 50 U/kg or FFP 15 mL/kg (if no concentrate available) & phytomenadione 10 mg IV (100 mcg/kg for children)
- INR > 4 & no active bleeding: PO Vitamin K (adult 10 mg daily and children 1-2.5 mg daily).

Poor INR control usually due to: medication noncompliance and/or low dietary Vitamin K intake or deficiency[4]

Management depends on: severity of INR elevation—presence of bleeding—thrombotic risk[5]

EVALUATION

INR

Consider CBC to assess anemia

Consider chemistry to assess renal function

MANAGEMENT

Warfarin supratherapeutic[7]:
- INR 4.5–10 with no bleeding—routine Vitamin K not recommended
- INR > 10 with no bleeding—po Vitamin K recommended
- Major bleeding—prothrombin complex concentrate & may use Vitamin K 5–10 mg slow IV

Heparin supratherapeutic[8]:
- (Note: no proven neutralization method if LMWH—protamine sulfate neutralizes anti-IIa activity)
- Protamine sulfate (dosing dependent on time since heparin infusion)
  - Minutes since infusion—1 mg per every 100 units of heparin

30 minutes—0.5 mg per every 100 units of heparin
> 120 minutes—0.25–0.375 mg per every 100 units of heparin
If heparin is given SQ:
1–1.5 mg per every 100 units of heparin
Load 25–50 mg slow IV, then remainder of dosing IV over 8–16 hours
INR supratherapeutic[9]:
≤5 (no bleeding)
Lower warfarin dose, or
Omit dose—resume at lower dose when INR therapeutic, or
No reduction if minimally supratherapeutic
>5–9 (no bleeding)
Omit next 1–2 doses, monitor INR, & resume at a lower dose, or
Omit dose & administer po Vitamin K 1–2.5 mg
>9 (no bleeding)
Hold warfarin & administer po vitamin K 2.5–5 mg
Monitor INR adding more Vitamin K if needed. Resume warfarin at a lower dose
Any INR level with serious bleeding
Hold warfarin. Administer Vitamin K 10 mg IV slowly. Supplement with prothrombin complex concentrate or FFP

Appendices

BURNS

Figure A.1 Estimating burn size accurately is essential for care of the burn patient. The rule of nines provides a simple algorithm for calculating the burned surface area. Reprinted with permission from Mulholland MW, Lillemoe KD, Doherty GM, Maier RV, Simeone DM, Upchurch GR, eds. *Greenfield's Surgery: Scientific Principles & Practice.* 5th ed. Philadelphia, PA: Lippincott Williams & Wilkins, 2011.

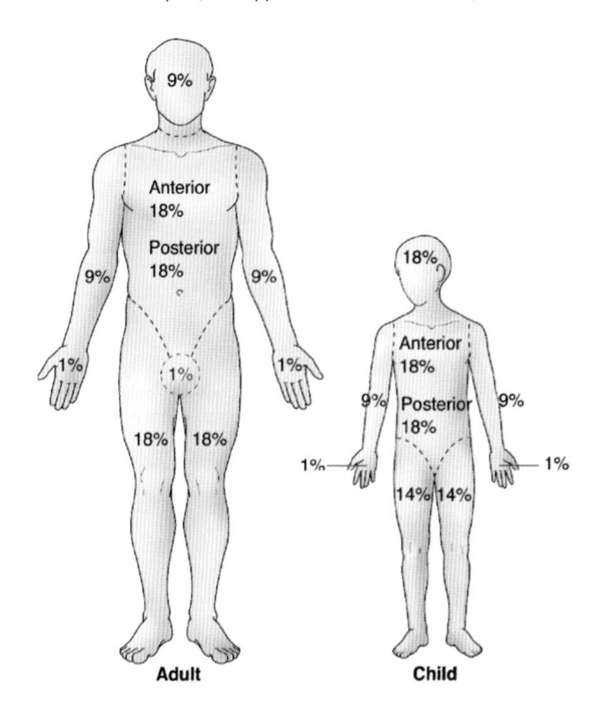

Table A.1 STD Treatment Summary

	CDC 2015 Guideline Summary
Bacterial vaginosis All regimens recommended for symptomatic pregnant females	Metronidazole 500 mg bid ×7 days or Clindamycin 300 mg bid ×7 days or Metronidazole gel 0.75% 5 g applicator HS ×5 days or Clindamycin cream 2% 5 g applicator HS ×7 days
Cervicitis/chlamydia Consider concurrent Tx for *N. gonorrhea*	Azithromycin 1 g PO single dose (*Ok in pregnancy*) or Doxycycline 100 mg bid 7 days or Levofloxin 500 mg daily ×7 days Amoxil 500 mg tid ×7 days (*Ok in pregnancy*)
Epididymitis	Ceftriaxone 250 mg IM single dose *plus* Doxycycline 100 mg bid ×10 days If enteric organism suspected (anal sex): Ceftriaxone 250 mg IM single dose *plus* Levofloxacin 500 mg daily ×10 days
Genital herpes simplex	Acyclovir 400 mg tid ×7-10 days or Valcyclovir 1 g bid ×7-10 days
Gonococcal infections	Ceftriaxone 250 mg IM single dose *plus* Azithromycin 1 g gram PO single dose
Lymphogranuloma venereum	Doxycycline 100 mg bid 21 days

CDC 2015 Guideline Summary	
Pediculosis pubis	Permethrin 1% cream rinse applied to area, wash off after 10 mins
Pelvic inflammatory Dz	Cefotetan 2 g IV bid *plus* doxycycline 100 mg po or IV bid or Ceftriaxone 250 mg IM single dose *plus* Doxycycline 100 mg bid 14 days Consider Metronidazole 500 mg bid ×14 days
Scabies	Permethrin 5% cream apply to body, wash off after 8 to 12 hours
Syphilis Primary/latent or early < 1 year	Benzathine penicillin G 2.4 million units IM single dose or Doxycycline 100 mg bid ×14 days
Latent > 1 year or unknown	Benzathine penicillin G 2.4 million units IM in 3 doses at 1-week intervals or Doxycycline 100 mg bid ×28 days
Trichomoniasis	Metronidazole 2 g PO single dose or 500 mg bid ×7 days ***Pregnant pts*** can be treated with 2 g single dose

From Morbidity and Mortality Weekly Report, *Recommendations and Reports*. 64:3. Centers for Disease Control and Prevention, 2015.

DERMATOME

Figure A.2 Dermatome map.

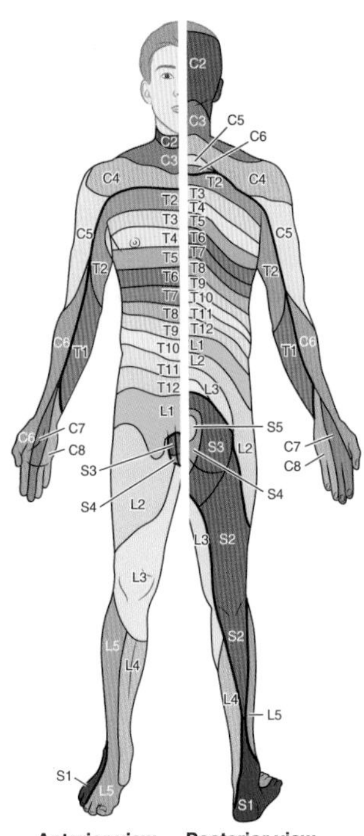

Reprinted with permission from Moore KL, Dalley AF, Agur AMR. *Clinically Oriented Anatomy*. 7th ed. Baltimore, MD: Lippincott Williams & Wilkins, 2014.

INSULIN SCALE

Table A.2 Sliding Scale Insulin Regimen

Blood Glucose, mg/dL	□ Insulin Sensitive	□ Usual	□ Insulin Resistant
> 141-180	2	4	6
181-220	4	6	8
221-260	6	8	10
261-300	8	10	12
301-350	10	12	14
351-400	12	14	16
> 400	14	16	18

Before meal: supplemental sliding scale insulin (number of units)—add to scheduled insulin dose; *bedtime*: give half of supplemental sliding scale insulin.

From Umpierrez GE, Smiley D, Zisman A, et al. Randomized study of basal-bolus insulin therapy in the inpatient management of patients with type 2 diabetes (RABBIT 2 trial). *Diabetes Care*. 2007;30(9):2181-2186.

MYOCARDIAL INFARCTION

Table A.3 Help With the Localization of a Myocardial Infarction (MI)

Localization	ST Elevation	Reciprocal ST Depression	Coronary Artery
Anterior MI	V_1-V_6	None	LAD
Septal MI	V_1-V_4, disappearance of septum Q in leads V_5, V_6	None	LAD-septal branches
Lateral MI	I, aVL, V_5, V_6	II, III, aVF	LCX or MO
Inferior MI	II, III, aVF	I, aVL	RCA (80%) or RCX (20%)
Posterior MI	V_7, V_8, V_9	high R in V_1-V_3 with ST depression V_1-V_3 > 2 mm (mirror view)	RCX
Right ventricle MI	V1, V_4R	I, aVL	RCA
Atrial MI	PTa in I, V_5, V_6	PTa in I, II, or III	RCA

ECG Criteria for STEMI

- New ST elevation
  - > 0.1 mV in 2 contiguous leads
  - Any 2 (II, III, aVF) or (v_2-v_6, I, aVL)
  - Not aVR or V1
- In V_2 & V_3
  - >=0.2 mV in men
  - >=0.15mV in women
- New LBBB

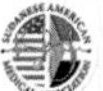

Thygsen et al. Universal Definition of MI
Circulation 2010

Data from Thygesen K, Alpert JS, Harvey D, White HD. Universal definition of myocardial infarction. *Circulation*. 2007;116:2634-2653.

PEDIATRIC VITALS

Table A.4 Normal Vital Signs for Age of Pediatric Patients

Age	Heart Rate, bpm	Respiratory Rate, bpm	Systolic Blood Pressure, mm Hg	Diastolic Blood Pressure, mm Hg
Newborn	90-180	30-50	60 ± 10	37 ± 10
1-5 months	100-180	30-40	80 ± 10	45 ± 15
6-11 months	100-150	25-35	90 ± 30	60 ± 10
1 yo	100-150	20-30	95 ± 30	65 ± 25
2-3 yo	65-150	15-25	100 ± 25	65 ± 25
4-5 yo	65-140	15-25	100 ± 20	65 ± 15
6-9 yo	65-120	12-20	100 ± 20	65 ± 15
10-12 yo	65-120	12-20	110 ± 20	70 ± 15
13+ yo	55-110	12-18	120 ± 20	75 ± 15

Adapted from Silverman BK. Practical Information. In: *Textbook of Pediatric Emergency Medicine*, 2006. Also: Jorden RC. Multiple Trauma. In: *Emergency Medicine: Concepts and Clinical Practice*, 1990.

SALTER HARRIS

Figure A.3 Salter-Harris classification. From Chowdhury S, Cozma A, Chowdhury J. *Essentials for the Canadian Medial Licensing Exam*. 2nd ed. St. Louis, MO: Wolters Kluwer Health, 2010.

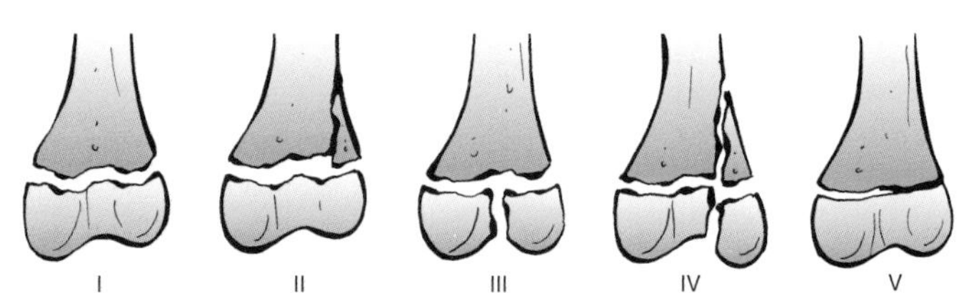

I = Physis
II = Metaphysis
III = Epiphysis
IV = ME (Metaphysis + Epiphysis) M+E = ME
V = Crush

WELLS SCORE

Table A.5 Wells Score (PE)

• Clinical signs and symptoms compatible with DVT	3
• PE judged to be the most likely diagnosis	3
• Surgery or bedridden for more than 3 days during past 4 weeks	1.5
• Previous DVT or PE	1.5
• Heart rate > 100 min^{-1}	1.5
• Hemoptysis	1
• Active cancer (treatment ongoing or within previous 6 months, or palliative treatment)	1

≤ 4: LOW (or "PE Unlikely") pretest probability; 4.5-6: MODERATE pretest probability; > 6: HIGH pretest probability.

Data from Wells PS, Anderson DR, Rodger M, et al. Derivation of a simple clinical model to categorize patients probability of pulmonary embolism: increasing the models utility with the SimpliRED D-dimer. *Thromb Haemost*. 2000;83:416-420; Kearon C, Ginsberg JS, Douketis J, et al. An evaluation of D-dimer in the diagnosis of pulmonary embolism. *Ann Intern Med*. 2006;144:812-821.

1. ABDOMINAL AORTIC ANEURYSM

1. Stather PW, Sidloff DA, Rhema IA, Choke E, Bown MJ, Sayers RD. A review of current reporting of abdominal aortic aneurysm mortality and prevalence in the literature. *Eur J Vasc Endovasc Surg*. 2014;47(3):240.
2. Johnston KW, Rutherford RB, Tilson MD, Shah DM, Hollier L, Stanley JC. Suggested standards for reporting on arterial aneurysms. Subcommittee on Reporting Standards for Arterial Aneurysms, Ad Hoc Committee on Reporting Standards, Society for Vascular Surgery and North American Chapter, International Society for Cardiovascular Surgery. *J Vasc Surg*. 1991;13(3):452.
3. Sweeting MJ, Thompson SG, Brown LC, Powell JT, RESCAN collaborators. Meta-analysis of individual patient data to examine factors affecting growth and rupture of small abdominal aortic aneurysms. *Br J Surg*. May 2012;99(5):655-665.
4. Kent KC, Zwolak RM, Egorova NN, et al. Analysis of risk factors for abdominal aortic aneurysm in a cohort of more than 3 million individuals. *J Vasc Surg*. 2010;52(3):539.
5. Rinckenbach S, Albertini JN, Thaveau F, et al. Prehospital treatment of infrarenal ruptured abdominal aortic aneurysms: a multicentric analysis. *Ann Vasc Surg*. 2010;24(3):308.
6. Marston WA, Ahlquist R, Johnson G Jr, Meyer AA. Misdiagnosis of ruptured abdominal aortic aneurysms. *J Vasc Surg*. 1992;16(1):17.
7. Mehta M, Taggert J, Darling RC III, et al. Establishing a protocol for endovascular treatment of ruptured abdominal aortic aneurysms: outcomes of a prospective analysis. *J Vasc Surg*. 2006;44(1):1.

2. ABDOMINAL PAIN

1. Yamamoto W, Kono H, Maekawa M, Fukui T. The relationship between abdominal pain regions and specific diseases: an epidemiologic approach to clinical practice. *J Epidemiol*. 1997;7(1):27.
2. Böhner H, Yang Q, Franke C, Verreet PR, Ohmann C. Simple data from history and physical examination help to exclude bowel obstruction and to avoid radiographic studies in patients with acute abdominal pain. *Eur J Surg*. 1998;164(10):777.
3. Bundy DG, Byerley JS, Liles EA, Perrin EM, Katznelson J, Rice HE. Does this child have appendicitis? *JAMA*. 25 July 2007;298(4):438-451.
4. Kessler N, Cyteval C, Gallix B, et al. Appendicitis: evaluation of sensitivity, specificity, and predictive values of US, Doppler US, and laboratory findings. *Radiology*. February 2004;230(2):472-478.
5. Hickey MS, Kiernan GJ, Weaver KE. Evaluation of abdominal pain. *Emerg Med Clin North Am*. August 1989;7(3):437-452.
6. Macaluso CR, McNamara RM. Evaluation and management of acute abdominal pain in the emergency department. *Int J Gen Med*. 2012;5:789-797.
7. Cartwright SL, Knudson MP. Evaluation of acute abdominal pain in adults. *Am Fam Physician*. 1 April 2008;77(7):971-978.

8. Manterola C, Vial M, Moraga J, Astudillo P. Analgesia in patients with acute abdominal pain. *Cochrane Database Syst Rev.* 19 January 2011;(1):CD005660.
9. Birnbaum A, Esses D, Bijur PE, Holden L, Gallagher EJ. Randomized double-blind placebo-controlled trial of two intravenous morphine dosages (0.10 mg/kg and 0.15 mg/kg) in emergency department patients with moderate to severe acute pain. *Ann Emerg Med.* April 2007;49(4):445-453.

3. ABG

1. Huttmann SE, Windisch W, Storre JH. Techniques for the measurement and monitoring of carbon dioxide in the blood. *Ann Am Thorac Soc.* May 2014;11(4):645-652.
2. American Association for Respiratory Care. AARC clinical practice guideline. Sampling for arterial blood gas analysis. *Respir Care.* August 1992;37(8):913-917.
3. Kelly A, McAlpine R, Kyle E. Venous pH can safely replace arterial pH in the initial evaluation of patients in the emergency department. *Emerg Med J.* September 2001;18(5):340-342.
4. Pramod S, Gunchan P, Sandeep P. Interpretation of arterial blood gas. *Indian J Crit Care Med.* April-June 2010;14(2):57-64.
5. Noh U-S, Yi J-H, Han S-W, Kim H-J. Varying dialysate bicarbonate concentrations in maintenance hemodialysis patients affect post-dialysis alkalosis but not pre-dialysis acidosis. *Electrolyte Blood Press.* December 2007; 5(2):95-101.
6. Bruno CM, Valenti M. Acid-base disorders in patients with chronic obstructive pulmonary disease: a pathophysiological review. *J Biomed Biotechnol.* 2012; 2012:915150.

4. ACETAMINOPHEN (APAP) OD

1. Lancaster EM, Hiatt JR, Zarrinpar A. Acetaminophen hepatotoxicity: an updated review. *Arch Toxicol.* February 2015;89(2):193-199.
2. Heard KJ. Acetylcysteine for acetaminophen poisoning. *N Engl J Med.* 17 July 2008;359(3):285-292.
3. Hodgman MJ, Garrard AR. A review of acetaminophen poisoning. *Crit Care Clin.* October 2012;28(4):499-516.
4. Blieden M, Paramore LC, Shah D, Ben-Joseph R. A perspective on the epidemiology of acetaminophen exposure and toxicity in the United States. *Expert Rev Clin Pharmacol.* May 2014;7(3):341-348.
5. Rumack BH. Acetaminophen hepatotoxicity: the first 35 years. *J Toxicol Clin Toxicol.* 2002;40(1):3-20.
6. Chun LJ, Tong MJ, Busuttil RW, Hiatt JR. Acetaminophen hepatotoxicity and acute liver failure. *J Clin Gastroenterol.* April 2009;43(4):342-349.
7. Mohler CR, Nordt SP, Williams SR, Manoguerra AS, Clark RF. Prospective evaluation of mild to moderate pediatric acetaminophen exposures. *Ann Emerg Med.* March 2000;35(3):239-244.

8. Yoon E, Babar A, Choudhary M, Kutner M, Pyrsopoulos N. Acetaminophen-induced hepatotoxicity: a comprehensive update. *J Clin Transl Hepatol.* 28 June 2016;4(2):131-142.
9. Brok J, Buckley N, Gluud C. Interventions for paracetamol (acetaminophen) overdose. *Cochrane Database Syst Rev.* 19 April 2006;(2):CD003328.
10. Spiller HA, Krenzelok EP, Grande GA, Safir EF, Diamond JJ. A prospective evaluation of the effect of activated charcoal before oral N-acetylcysteine in acetaminophen overdose. *Ann Emerg Med.* March 1994;23(3):519-523.
11. Buckley NA, Whyte IM, O'Connell DL, Dawson AH. Activated charcoal reduces the need for N-acetylcysteine treatment after acetaminophen (paracetamol) overdose. *J Toxicol Clin Toxicol.* 1999;37(6):753.
12. Smilkstein MJ, Bronstein AC, Linden C, Augenstein WL, Kulig KW, Rumack BH. Acetaminophen overdose: a 48-hour intravenous N-acetylcysteine treatment protocol. *Ann Emerg Med.* 1991;20(10):1058.
13. Wang GS, Monte A, Bagdure D, Heard K. Hepatic failure despite early acetylcysteine following large acetaminophen-diphenhydramine overdose. *Pediatrics.* April 2011;127(4):e1077-e1080.
14. Green JL, Heard KJ, Reynolds KM, Albert D. Oral and intravenous acetylcysteine for treatment of acetaminophen toxicity: a systematic review and meta-analysis. *West J Emerg Med.* 2013;14(3):218.
15. Riggs BS, Bronstein AC, Kulig K, Archer PG, Rumack BH. Acute acetaminophen overdose during pregnancy. *Obstet Gynecol.* 1989;74(2):247.

5. ACLS

1. American Heart Association. Adult advanced cardiovascular life support: 2010. American Heart Association guidelines for cardiopulmonary resuscitation and emergency cardiovascular care. *Circulation.* 2 November 2010;122(18):S3.

6. ACLS GENERAL

1. Valenzuela TD, Kern KB, Clark LL, et al. Interruptions of chest compressions during emergency medical systems resuscitation. *Circulation.* 2005;112(9):1259.
2. International Liaison Committee on Resuscitation. 2005 International consensus on cardiopulmonary resuscitation and emergency cardiovascular care science with treatment recommendations. Part 2: Adult basic life support. *Resuscitation.* 2005;67(2-3):187.
3. Hasegawa K, Hiraide A, Chang Y, Brown DFM. Association of prehospital advanced airway management with neurologic outcome and survival in patients with out-of-hospital cardiac arrest. *JAMA.* 2013;309(3):257.
4. Van Walraven C, Forster AJ, Stiell IG. Derivation of a clinical decision rule for the discontinuation of in-hospital cardiac arrest resuscitations. *Arch Intern Med.* 25 Januray 1999;159(2):129-134.

5. Jabre P, Bougouin W, Dumas F, et al. Early identification of patients with out-of-hospital cardiac arrest with no chance of survival and consideration for organ donation. *Ann Intern Med.* 6 December 2016;165(11):770-778.

7. ACUTE CORONARY SYNDROME

1. Amsterdam EA, Wenger NK, Brindis RG, et al. 2014 AHA/ACC guideline for the management of patients with non-ST-elevation Acute Coronary Syndromes: a report of the American College of Cardiology/American Heart Association Task Force on practice guidelines. *J Am Coll Cardiol.* 23 December 2014;64(24):e139-e228.
2. Braunwald E. Unstable angina and non-ST elevation myocardial infarction. *Am J Respir Crit Care Med.* 1 May 2012;185(9):924-932.
3. Mant J, McManus RJ, Oakes RA, et al. Systematic review and modelling of the investigation of acute and chronic chest pain presenting in primary care. *Health Technol Assess.* February 2004;8(2):iii; 1-158.
4. Goodacre S, Locker T, Morris F, Campbell S. How useful are clinical features in the diagnosis of acute, undifferentiated chest pain? *Acad Emerg Med.* March 2002;9(3):203-208.
5. Amsterdam EA, Wenger NK, Brindis RG, et al. 2014 AHA/ACC guideline for the management of patients with non-ST-elevation acute coronary syndromes: a report of the American College of Cardiology/American Heart Association Task Force on practice guidelines. *Circulation.* 23 December 2014;130(25):e344-e426.
6. Antman EM, Anbe DT, Armstrong PW, et al. ACC/AHA guidelines for the management of patients with ST-elevation myocardial infarction: a report of the American College of Cardiology/American Heart Association task force on practice guidelines (Committee to Revise the 1999 Guidelines for the Management of Patients with Acute Myocardial Infarction). *Circulation.* 31 August 2004;110(9):e82-e292.
7. O'Gara PT, Kushner FG, Ascheim DD, et al. 2013 ACCF/AHA guideline for the management of ST-elevation myocardial infarction: a report of the American College of Cardiology Foundation/American Heart Association Task Force on practice guidelines. *Circulation.* 2013;127(4):e362.
8. Shuvy M, Atar D, Gabriel Steg P, et al. Oxygen therapy in acute coronary syndrome: are the benefits worth the risk? *Eur Heart J.* 2013;34(22):1630.
9. Cabello JB, Burls A, Emparanza JI, Bayliss S, Quinn T. Oxygen therapy for acute myocardial infarction. *Cochrane Database Syst Rev.* 21 August 2013;(8):CD007160.
10. Goyal A, Spertus JA, Gosch K, et al. Serum potassium levels and mortality in acute myocardial infarction. *JAMA.* January 2012;307(2):157-164.

8. ACUTE LOW BACK PAIN (LBP)

1. Husband DJ. Malignant spinal cord compression: prospective study of delays in referral and treatment. *BMJ.* 1998;317(7150):18.
2. Chou R. In the clinic: low back pain. *Ann Intern Med.* June 2014;160(11):ITC6-1.

3. Helweg-Larsen S, Sørensen PS. Symptoms and signs in metastatic spinal cord compression: a study of progression from first symptom until diagnosis in 153 patients. *Eur J Cancer.* 1994;30A(3):396.
4. Chen WC, Wang JL, Wang JT, Chen YC, Chang SC. Spinal epidural abscess due to staphylococcus aureus: clinical manifestations and outcomes. *J Microbiol Immunol Infect.* 2008;41(3):215.
5. Darouiche RO, Hamill RJ, Greenberg SB, Weathers SW, Musher DM. Bacterial spinal epidural abscess. Review of 43 cases and literature survey. *Medicine* (Baltimore). 1992;71(6):369.
6. Deyo RA, Diehl AK. Cancer as a cause of back pain: frequency, clinical presentation, and diagnostic strategies. *J Gen Intern Med.* 1988;3(3):230.
7. Davis DP, Salazar A, Chan TC, Vilke GM. Prospective evaluation of a clinical decision guideline to diagnose spinal epidural abscess in patients who present to the emergency department with spine pain. *J Neurosurg Spine.* 2011;14(6):765.
8. Reihsaus E, Waldbaur H, Seeling W. Spinal epidural abscess: a meta-analysis of 915 patients. *Neurosurg Rev.* December 2000;23(4):175-204.
9. Chou R, Fu R, Carrino JA, Deyo RA. Imaging strategies for low-back pain: systematic review and meta-analysis. *Lancet.* 2009;373(9662):463.
10. Chou R, Qaseem A, Snow V, et al. Diagnosis and treatment of low back pain: a joint clinical practice guideline from the American College of Physicians and the American Pain Society. Clinical Efficacy Assessment Subcommittee of the American College of Physicians, American College of Physicians, American Pain Society Low Back Pain Guidelines Panel. *Ann Intern Med.* 2007;147(7):478.
11. Apeldoorn AT, Bosselaar H, Blom-Luberti T, Twisk JW, Lankhorst GJ. The reliability of nonorganic sign-testing and the Waddell score in patients with chronic low back pain. *Spine* (Phila Pa 1976). 1 April 2008;33(7):821-826.
12. Kumar N, Wijerathne SI, Lim WW, Barry TW, Nath C, Liang S. Resistive straight leg raise test, resistive forward bend test, and heel compression test: novel techniques in identifying secondary gain motives in low back pain cases. *Eur Spine J.* November 2012;21(11):2280-2286.
13. Koes BW, Van Tulder MW, Thomas S. Diagnosis and treatment of low back pain. *BMJ.* 17 June 2006;332(7555):1430.
14. Kinkade S. Evaluation and treatment of acute low back pain. *Am Fam Physician.* 15 April 2007;75(8):1181-1188.

9. ALCOHOL WITHDRAWAL

1. Brousse G, Arnaud B, Vorspan F, et al. Alteration of glutamate/GABA balance during acute alcohol withdrawal in emergency department: a prospective analysis. *Alcohol Alcohol.* September-October 2012;47(5):501-508.
2. Etherington JM. Emergency management of acute alcohol problems. Part 1: uncomplicated withdrawal. *Can Fam Physician.* 1996;42:2186.

3. Victor M, Brausch C. The role of abstinence in the genesis of alcoholic epilepsy. *Epilepsia.* 1967;8(1):1.
4. Sechi G, Serra A. Wernicke's encephalopathy: new clinical settings and recent advances in diagnosis and management. *Lancet Neurol.* May 2007;6(5):442-455.
5. Ferguson JA, Suelzer CJ, Eckert GJ, Zhou XH, Dittus RS. Risk factors for delirium tremens development. *J Gen Intern Med.* 1996;11(7):410.
6. Smith MF, Beecher LH, Fischer TL, et al. Management of alcohol withdrawal delirium. An evidence-based practice guideline. *Arch Intern Med.* 2004;164(13):1405.
7. Hack JB, Hoffman RS. Thiamine before glucose to prevent Wernicke encephalopathy: examining the conventional wisdom. *JAMA.* 1998;279(8):583.
8. Wilson A, Vulcano B. A double-blind, placebo-controlled trial of magnesium sulfate in the ethanol withdrawal syndrome. *Alcohol Clin Exp Resp.* 1984;8:542-545.
9. Saitz R, Mayo-Smith MF, Roberts MS, Redmond HA, Bernard DR, Calkins DR. Individualized treatment for alcohol withdrawal. A randomized double-blind controlled trial. *JAMA.* 17 August 1994;272(7):519-523.
10. Amato L, Minozzi S, Davoli M. Efficacy and safety of pharmacological interventions for the treatment of the alcohol withdrawal syndrome. *Cochrane Database Syst Rev.* 15 June 2011;(6):CD008537.
11. Jaeger TM, Lohr RH, Pankratz VS. Symptom-triggered therapy for alcohol withdrawal syndrome in medical inpatients. *Mayo Clin Proc.* 2001;76(7):695.
12. Rathlev NK, D'Onofrio G, Fish SS, et al. The lack of efficacy of phenytoin in the prevention of recurrent alcohol-related seizures. *Ann Emerg Med.* March 1994;23(3):513-518.
13. Hack JB, Hoffmann RS, Nelson LS. Resistant alcohol withdrawal: does an unexpectedly large sedative requirement identify these patients early? *J Med Toxicol.* 2006;2(2):55.
14. Rosenson J, Clements C, Simon B, et al. Phenobarbital for acute alcohol withdrawal: a prospective randomized double-blind placebo-controlled study. *J Emerg Med.* March 2013;44(3):592-598.
15. McCowan C, Marik P. Refractory delirium tremens treated with propofol: a case series. *Crit Care Med.* 2000;28(6):1781.
16. Blum K, Eubanks JD, Wallace JE, Hamilton H. Enhancement of alcohol withdrawal convulsions in mice by haloperidol. *Clin Toxicol.* 1976;9(3):427.
17. Blondell RD. Ambulatory detoxification of patients with alcohol dependence. *Am Fam Physician.* 2005;71(3):495.

10. ANGIOEDEMA

1. Moellman JJ, Bernstein JA, Lindsell C, et al. A consensus parameter for the evaluation and management of angioedema in the emergency department. *Acad Emerg Med.* April 2014;21(4):469-484.
2. Caballero T, Baeza ML, Cabañas R, et al. Consensus statement on the diagnosis, management, and treatment of angioedema mediated by bradykinin. Part II.

Treatment, follow-up, and special situations. *J Investig Allergol Clin Immunol.* 2011;21(6):422-441.
3. Greaves MW, Sabroe RA. ABC of allergies. Allergy and the skin. I-xUrticaria. *BMJ.* 1998;316(7138):1147.
4. Bas M, Hoffmann TK, Bier H, Kojda G. Increased C-reactive protein in ACE-inhibitor-induced angioedema. *Br J Clin Pharmacol.* February 2005;59(2):233-238.
5. Scheirey CD, Scholz FJ, Shortsleeve MJ, Katz DS. Angiotensin-converting enzyme inhibitor-induced small-bowel angioedema: clinical and imaging findings in 20 patients. *AJR Am J Roentgenol.* August 2011;197(2):393-398.
6. Arakawa M, Murata Y, Rikimaru Y, Sasaki Y. Drug-induced isolated visceral angioneurotic edema. *Intern Med.* 2005;44(9):975.
7. Simons FE. Emergency treatment of anaphylaxis. *BMJ.* 2008;336(7654):1141.

11. ANKLE/FOOT/KNEE

1. Stiell IG, Greenberg GH, McKnight RD, et al. Decision rules for the use of radiography in acute ankle injuries. Refinement and prospective validation. *JAMA.* 3 March 1993;269(9):1127-1132.
2. Hawley C, Rosenblatt R. Ottawa and Pittsburgh rules for acute knee injuries. *J Fam Pract.* October 1998;47(4):254-255.
3. Seaberg DC, Yealy DM, Lukens T, Auble T, Mathias S. Multicenter comparison of two clinical decision rules for the use of radiography in acute, high-risk knee injuries. *Ann Emerg Med.* July 1998;32(1):8-13.

12. ANXIETY DISORDER

1. American Psychiatric Association. *Diagnostic and Statistical Manual of Mental Disorders,* 5th ed. Virginia, VA: American Psychiatric Association; 2013.
2. Katzman MA, Bleau P, Blier P, et al. Canadian anxiety guidelines initiative group. *BMC Psychiatry.* 2014;14 (1 suppl):S1.
3. Hoge EA, Ivkovic A, Fricchione GL. Generalized anxiety disorder: diagnosis and treatment. *BMJ.* 27 November 2012;345:e7500.
4. Herr N, Williams J, Benjamin S, McDuffie J. Does this patient have generalized anxiety or panic disorder?: the Rational Clinical Examination systematic review. *JAMA.* 2 July 2014;312(1):78.
5. Hamilton M. The assessment of anxiety states by rating. *Br J Med Psychol.* 1959;32(1):50-55.
6. Offidani E, Guidi J, Tomba E, Fava GA. Efficacy and tolerability of benzodiazepines versus antidepressants in anxiety disorders: a systematic review and meta-analysis. *Psychother Psychosom.* 2013;82(6):355-362.
7. Guaiana G, Barbui C, Cipriani A. Hydroxyzine for generalised anxiety disorder. *Cochrane Database Syst Rev.* 8 December 2010;(12):CD006815.

8. Citrome L. Comparison of intramuscular ziprasidone, olanzapine, or aripiprazole for agitation: a quantitative review of efficacy and safety. *J Clin Psychiatry.* December 2007;68(12):1876-1885.
9. Calver L, Drinkwater V, Gupta R, Page CB, Isbister GK. Droperidol v. haloperidol for sedation of aggressive behavior in acute mental health: randomised controlled trial. *Br J Psychiatry.* 2015;206(3):223.
10. Stein BM, Goin KM, Pollack HM, et al. Practice guideline for the treatment of patients with panic disorder. In, Fochtmann L.J., ed. *American Psychiatric Association.* January 2009. www.aafp.org/afp
11. Riddell J, Tran A, Bengiamin R, Hendey GW, Armenian P. Ketamine as a first-line treatment for severely agitated emergency department patients. *Am J Emerg Med.* 2017;35(7):1000-1004.

13. ASTHMA

1. National Asthma Education and Prevention Program. Expert Panel Report 3 (EPR-3): guidelines for the diagnosis and management of asthma-summary report 2007. *J Allergy Clin Immunol.* November 2007;120(5 Suppl):S94-S138.
2. Goodacre S, Bradburn M, Cohen J, et al. Prediction of unsuccessful treatment in patients with severe acute asthma. *Emerg Med J.* October 2014;31(e1):e40-e45.
3. U.S. Department of Health and Human Services. *Guidelines for the diagnosis and management of asthma.* National Heart, Lung, and Blood Institute; [2007; cited 15 May 2017]. https://www.nhlbi.nih.gov/files/docs/guidelines/asthgdln.pdf.
4. Kelsen SG, Kelsen DP, Fleeger BF, Jones RC, Rodman T. Emergency room assessment and treatment of patients with acute asthma. Adequacy of the conventional approach. *Am J Med.* 1978;64(4):622.
5. Nowak RM, Tomlanovich MC, Sarkar DD, Kvale PA, Anderson JA. Arterial blood gases and pulmonary function testing in acute bronchial asthma. Predicting patient outcomes. *JAMA.* 1983;249(15):2043.
6. British Thoracic Society. British guideline on the management of asthma. *Thorax.* 2014;69 (1 Suppl):1.
7. Normansell R, Kew KM, Mansour G. Different oral corticosteroid regimens for acute asthma. *Cochrane Database Syst Rev.* 13 May 2016;(5):CD011801.
8. Carroll CL. Just a lot of hot air? Volatile anesthetics in children with status asthmaticus. *Pediatr Crit Care Med.* May 2013;14(4):433-434.
9. Johnston SL, Szigeti M, Cross M, et al. Azithromycin for acute exacerbations of asthma: the AZALEA randomized clinical trial. *JAMA Intern Med.* 2016;176(11):1630.

14. BACKBOARD CLEARANCE

1. Brown LH, Gough JE, Simonds WB. Can EMS providers adequately assess trauma patients for cervical spinal injury? *Prehosp Emerg Care.* 1998;2(1):33.

2. Oteir AO, Smith K, Stoelwinder JU, Middleton J, Jennings PA. Should suspected cervical spinal cord injury be immobilized?: a systematic review. *Injury.* April 2015;46(4):528-535.
3. Totten VY, Sugarman DB. Respiratory effects of spinal immobilization. *Prehosp Emerg Care.* October-December 1999;3(4):347-352.
4. Cordell WH, Hollingsworth JC, Olinger ML, Stroman SJ, Nelson DR. Pain and tissue interface pressures during spine board immobilization. *Acad Emerg Med.* 1995;26:31-36.
5. Cooney DR, Wallus H, Asaly M, Wojcik S. Backboard time for patients receiving spinal immobilization by emergency medical services. *Int J Emerg Med.* 20 June 2013;6:17.
6. Sutcliffe AJ. Spinal cord injury and direct laryngoscopy—the legend lives on. *Br J Anaesth.* 2000;85(4):665.
7. Michaleff ZA, Maher CG, Verhagen AP, Rebbeck T, Lin CW. Accuracy of the Canadian C-spine rule and NEXUS to screen for clinically important cervical spine injury in patients following blunt trauma: a systematic review. *Can Med Assoc J.* 2012;184:867-876.
8. Mathen R, Inaba K, Munera F, et al. Prospective evaluation of multislice computed tomography versus plain radiographic cervical spine clearance in trauma patients. *J Trauma Inj Infect Crit Care.* 2007;62:1427-1431.
9. Como JJ, Diaz JJ, Dunham CM, et al. Practice management guidelines for identification of cervical spine injuries following trauma: update from the Eastern Association for the Surgery of Trauma Practice Management Guidelines Committee. *J Trauma.* 2009;67:651-659.
10. Milby AH, Halpern CH, Guo W, Stein SC. Prevalence of cervical spinal injury in trauma. *Neurosurg Focus.* 2008;25(5):E10.

15. BELL'S PALSY

1. Gilden DH. Clinical practice. Bell's palsy. *N Engl J Med.* 23 September 2004;351(13):1323-1331.
2. Fahimi J, Navi BB, Kamel H. Potential misdiagnoses of Bell's palsy in the emergency department. *Ann Emerg Med.* 2014;63(4):428.
3. Holland NJ, Weiner GM. Recent developments in Bell's Palsy. *BMJ.* 4 September 2004;329(7465):553-557.
4. American College of Radiology. ACR appropriateness criteria for cranial neuropathy. *J Am Coll Rad.* November 2017;14(11):S406-S420.
5. Jain V, Dishmukh A, Gollomp S. Bilateral facial paralysis: case presentations and discussion of differential diagnosis. *J Gen Intern Med.* July 2006;21(7):C7-C10.
6. Gronseth GS, Paduga R. Evidence-based guideline update: steroids and antivirals for Bell palsy: report of the Guideline Development Subcommittee of the American Academy of Neurology. American Academy of Neurology. *Neurology.* 2012;79(22):2209.
7. Baugh RF, Basura GH, Ishii LE, et al. American Academy of Otolaryngology-Head and Neck Surgery Foundation clinical guideline on Bell's Palsy. *Otolaryngol Head Neck Surg.* November 2013;149(3 Suppl):S1-S27.
8. Vrabec JT, Isaacson B, Van Hook JW. Bell's Palsy and pregnancy. *Otolaryngol Head Neck Surg.* December 2007;137(6):858-861.

9. Cohen Y, Lavie O, Granovsky-Grisaru S, Aboulafia Y, Diamant YZ. Bell Palsy complication pregnancy: a review. *Obstet Gynecol Surv.* March 2000; 55(3):184-188.

16. BRONCHITIS

1. Wenzel RP, Fowler AA III. Clinical practice. Acute bronchitis. *N Engl J Med.* 2006;355(20):2125.
2. Altiner A, Wilm S, Däubener W, et al. Sputum colour for diagnosis of a bacterial infection in patients with acute cough. *Scand J Prim Health Care.* 2009;27(2):70-73.
3. Clark TW, Medina MJ, Batham S, Curran MD, Parmar S, Nicholson KG. Adults hospitalised with acute respiratory illness rarely have detectable bacteria in the absence of COPD or pneumonia; viral infection predominates in a large prospective UK sample. *J Infect.* 2014;69(5):507.
4. Bushyhead JB, Wood RW, Tompkins RK, Wolcott BW, Diehr P. The effect of chest radiographs on the management and clinical course of patients with acute cough. *Med Care.* 1983;21(7):661.
5. Gonzales R, Bartlett JG, Besser RE, et al. Principles of appropriate antibiotic use for treatment of uncomplicated acute bronchitis: background. *Ann Intern Med.* 2001;134(6):521.
6. Schuetz P, Christ-Crain M, Thomann R, et al. Effect of procalcitonin-based guidelines vs standard guidelines on antibiotic use in lower respiratory tract infections: the ProHOSP randomized controlled trial. *JAMA.* 9 September 2009;302(10):1059-1066.
7. Wenzel RP, Fowler AA III. Clinical practice. Acute bronchitis. *N Engl J Med.* 16 November 2006;355(20):2125-2130.
8. Brown MO, St Anna L, Ohl M. Clinical inquiries. What are the indications for evaluating a patient with cough for pertussis? *J Fam Pract.* January 2005;54(1):74-76.
9. Centers for Disease Control and Prevention. Recommended antimicrobial agents for the treatment and postexposure prophylaxis of pertussis. 2005 CDC guidelines. *MMWR.* 2005;54:10.
10. King DE, Williams WC, Bishop L, Shechter A. Effectiveness of erythromycin in the treatment of acute bronchitis. *J Fam Pract.* June 1996;42(6):601-605.
11. Harris AM, Hicks LA, Qaseem A. Appropriate antibiotic use for acute respiratory tract infection in adults: advice for high-value care from the American College of Physicians and the Centers for Disease Control and Prevention. *Ann Intern Med.* 15 March 2016;164(6):425-434.
12. Hueston WJ. Albuterol delivered by metered-dose inhaler to treat acute bronchitis. *J Fam Pract.* November 1994;39(5):437-440.

17. CARBON MONOXIDE TOXICITY

1. Ginsberg MD. Carbon monoxide intoxication: clinical features, neuropathology, and mechanisms of injury. *J Toxicol Clin Toxicol.* 1985;23(4-6):281-288.
2. Ernst A, Zibrak JD. Carbon monoxide poisoning. *N Engl J Med.* 1998;339(22):1603.

3. Yasuda H, Yamaya M, Nakayama K, et al. Increased arterial carboxyhemoglobin concentrations in chronic obstructive pulmonary disease. *Am J Respir Crit Care Med.* 2005;171(11):1246.
4. Mégarbane B, Delahaye A, Goldgran-Tolédano D, Baud FJ.. Antidotal treatment of cyanide poisoning. *J Chin Med Assoc.* April 2003;66(4):193-203.
5. Weaver LK, Howe S, Hopkins R, Chan KJ. Carboxyhemoglobin half-life in carbon monoxide-poisoned patients treated with 100% oxygen at atmospheric pressure. *Chest.* March 2000;117(3):801-808.
6. Tomaszewski C. Carbon monoxide poisoning. Early awareness and intervention can save lives. *Postgrad Med.* 1999;105(1):39.
7. Harper A, Croft-Baker J. Carbon monoxide poisoning: undetected by both patients and their doctors. *Age Ageing.* 2004;33(2):105.
8. Thom SR, Taber RL, Mendiguren II, Clark JM, Hardy KR, Fisher AB. Delayed neuropsychologic sequelae after carbon monoxide poisoning: prevention by treatment with hyperbaric oxygen. *Ann Emerg Med.* 1995;25(4):474.
9. Satran D, Henry CR, Adkinson C, Nicholson CI, Bracha Y, Henry TD. Cardiovascular manifestations of moderate to severe carbon monoxide poisoning. *J Am Coll Cardiol.* 2005;45(9):1513.
10. Bozeman WP, Myers RA, Barish RA. Confirmation of the pulse oximetry gap in carbon monoxide poisoning. *Ann Emerg Med.* 1997;30(5):608.
11. Touger M, Gallagher EJ, Tyrell J. Relationship between venous and arterial carboxyhemoglobin levels in patients with suspected carbon monoxide poisoning. *Ann Emerg Med.* April 1995;25(4):481-483.
12. DiDonna TA Jr. Carbon monoxide poisoning. *Nursing.* January 1997;27(1):33.
13. Kao LW, Nañagas KA. Carbon monoxide poisoning. *Emerg Med Clin North Am.* 2004;22(4):985.
14. Hampson NB, Piantadosi CA, Thom SR, Weaver LK. Practice recommendations in the diagnosis, management, and prevention of carbon monoxide poisoning. *Am J Respir Crit Care Med.* 1 December 2012;186(11):1095-1101.

18. CELLULITIS

1. Swartz MN. Clinical practice. Cellulitis. *N Engl J Med.* 26 February 2004;350(9):904-912.
2. Raff AB, Kroshinsky D. Cellulitis: a review. *JAMA.* July 2016;316(3):325-337.
3. Bernard P, Bedane C, Mounier M, Denis F, Catanzano G, Bonnetblanc JM. Streptococcal cause of erysipelas and cellulitis in adults. A microbiologic study using a direct immunofluorescence technique. *Arch Dermatol.* 1989;125(6):779.
4. Jeng A, Beheshti M, Li J, Nathan R. The role of beta-hemolytic streptococci in causing diffuse, nonculturable cellulitis: a prospective investigation. *Medicine* (Baltimore). 2010;89(4):217.
5. Perl B, Gottehrer NP, Raveh D, Schlesinger Y, Rudensky B, Yinnon AM. Cost-effectiveness of blood cultures for adult patients with cellulitis. *Clin Infect Dis.* 1999;29(6):1483.

6. Stevens DL, Bison AL, Chambers HF. Practice guidelines for the diagnosis and management of skin and soft-tissue infections. *Clin Infect Dis.* 15 November 2005;41(10):1373-1406.
7. Thomas KS, Crook AM, Nunn AJ, et al. Penicillin to prevent recurrent leg cellulitis. U.K. Dermatology Clinical Trials Network's PATCH I Trial Team. *N Engl J Med.* May 2013;368(18):1695-1703.
8. Klempner MS, Styrt B. Prevention of recurrent staphylococcal skin infections with low-dose oral clindamycin therapy. *JAMA.* 1988;260(18):2682.
9. Aboltins CA, Hutchinson AF, Sinnappu RN. Oral versus parenteral antimicrobials for the treatment of cellulitis: a randomized non-inferiority trial. *J Antimicrob Chemother.* February 2015;70(2):581-586.
10. Sabbaj A, Jensen B, Browning MA. Soft tissue infections and emergency department disposition: predicting the need for inpatient admission. *Acad Emerg Med.* December 2009;16(12):1290-1297.
11. Claeys KC, Lagnf AM, Patel TB, Jacob MG, Davis SL, Rybak MJ. Acute bacterial skin and skin structure infections treated with intravenous antibiotics in the emergency department or observational unit: experience at the Detroit Medical Center. *Infect Dis Ther.* June 2015; 4(2):173-186.
12. Stevens DL, Bisno AL, Chambers HF, et al. Practice guidelines for the diagnosis and management of skin and soft tissue infections: 2014 update by the Infectious Diseases Society of America. *Clin Infect Di.* 2014;59(2):e10.
13. Rajendran PM, Young D, Maurer T, et al. Randomized, double-blind, placebo-controlled trial of cephalexin for treatment of uncomplicated skin abscesses in a population at risk for community-acquired methicillin-resistant staphylococcus aureus infection. *Antimicrob Agents Chemother.* 2007;51(11):4044.

19. COPD

1. Buist AS, McBurnie MA, Vollmer WM, et al. International variation in the prevalence of COPD (the BOLD Study): a population-based prevalence study. *Lancet.* 2007;370(9589):741.
2. Stoller JK, Aboussouan LS. Alpha1-antitrypsin deficiency. *Lancet.* 2005; 365(9478): 2225-2236.
3. From the Global Strategy for the Diagnosis, Management and Prevention of COPD, Global Initiative for Chronic Obstructive Lung Disease (GOLD) 2017. http://goldcopd.org.
4. Rennard S, Decramer M, Calverley PM, et al. Impact of COPD in North America and Europe in 2000: subjects' perspective of Confronting COPD International Survey. *Eur Respir J.* 2002;20(4):799.
5. Badgett RG, Tanaka DJ, Hunt DK, et al. Can moderate chronic obstructive pulmonary disease be diagnosed by historical and physical findings alone? *Am J Med.* 1993;94(2):188.
6. Brusasco V, Martinez F. Chronic obstructive pulmonary disease. *Compr Physiol.* January 2014;4(1):1-31.

7. Kelly AM, McAlpine R, Kyle E. How accurate are pulse oximeters in patients with acute exacerbations of chronic obstructive airways disease? *Respir Med.* 2001;95(5):336.
8. Seemungal TA, Wilkinson TM, Hurst JR, Perera WR, Sapsford RJ, Wedzicha JA. Long-term erythromycin therapy is associated with decreased chronic obstructive pulmonary disease exacerbations. *Am J Respir Crit Care Med.* 2008;178(11):1139.
9. Puhan MA, Vollenweider D, Latshang T, Steurer J, Steurer-Stey C. Exacerbations of chronic obstructive pulmonary disease: when are antibiotics indicated? A systematic review. *Respir Res.* 4 April 2007;8:30.
10. Vollenweider DJ, Jarrett H, Steurer-Stey CA, Garcia-Aymerich J, Puhan MA. Antibiotics for exacerbations of chronic obstructive pulmonary disease. *Cochrane Database Syst Rev.* 12 December 2012;12:CD010257.
11. Rodrigo G, Pollack C, Rodrigo C, Rowe B. Heliox for treatment of exacerbations of chronic obstructive pulmonary disease. *Cochrane Database Syst Rev.* 2002;(2):CD003571.
12. Skorodin MS, Tenholder MF, Yetter B, et al. Magnesium sulfate in exacerbations of chronic obstructive pulmonary disease. *Arch Intern Med.* 13 March 1995;155(5):496-500.
13. Khan SY, O'Driscoll BR. Is nebulized saline a placebo in COPD? *BMC Pulm Med.* 30 September 2004;4:9.

20. CORNEAL ABRASION

1. Wipperman JL, Dorsch JN. Evaluation and management of corneal abrasions. *Am Fam Physician.* 15 January 2013;87(2):114-120.
2. Arey ML, Mootha VV, Whittemore AR, Chason DP, Blomquist PH. Computed tomography in the diagnosis of occult open-globe injuries. *Ophthalmology.* 2007;114(8):1448.
3. Brandt MT, Haug RH. Traumatic hyphema: a comprehensive review. *J Oral Maxillofac Surg.* 2001;59(12):1462.
4. Ahmed F, House RJ, Feldman BH. Corneal abrasions and corneal foreign bodies. *Prim Care.* September 2015;42(3):363-375.
5. Waldman N, Winrow B, Densie I, et al. An observational study to determine whether routinely sending patients home with a 24-hour supply of topical tetracaine from the Emergency Department for simple corneal abrasion pain is potentially safe. *Ann Emerg Med.* 2 May 2017;pii: S0196-0644(17)30195-30196.
6. Waldman N, Densie IK, Herbison P. Topical tetracaine used for 24 hours is safe and rated highly effective by patients for the treatment of pain caused by corneal abrasions: a double-blind, randomized clinical trial. *Acad Emerg Med.* April 2014;21(4):374-382.
7. Dargin JM, Lowenstein RA. The painful eye. *Emerg Med Clin North Am.* February 2008;26(1):199-216, viii.
8. Calder LA, Balasubramanian S, Fergusson D. Topical nonsteroidal anti-inflammatory drugs for corneal abrasions: meta-analysis of randomized trials. *Acad Emerg Med.* May 2005;12(5):467-473.

21. CROUP

1. Peltola V, Heikkinen T, Ruuskanen O. Clinical courses of croup caused by influenza and parainfluenza viruses. *Pediatr Infect Dis J.* 2002;21(1):76.
2. Bjornson CL, Johnson DW. Croup. *Lancet.* 2008;371(9609):329.
3. Clarke M, Allaire J. An evidence-based approach to the evaluation and treatment of croup in children. *Pediatr Emerg Med Pract.* 2012;9(9):1.
4. Mills JL, Spackman TJ, Borns P, Mandell GA, Schwartz W. The usefulness of lateral neck roentgenograms in laryngotracheobronchitis. *Am J Dis Child.* 1979;133(11):1140.
5. Cherry JD. Clinical practice. Croup. *N Engl J Med.* 24 January 2008;358(4):384-391.
6. Denny FW, Clyde WA Jr. Acute lower respiratory tract infections in nonhospitalized children. *J Pediatr.* 1986;108(5 Pt 1):635.
7. Alberta Medical Association. *Guideline for the diagnosis and management of croup.* [Internet]. University of Washington [updated January 2008; cited 15 June 2017]. http://media.hsl.washington.edu/media/safranek/fpin/croup-guideline.pdf.
8. Petrocheilou A, Tanou K, Kalampouka E, Malakasioti G, Giannios C, Kaditis AG. Viral croup: diagnosis and a treatment algorithm. *Pediatr Pulmonol.* May 2014;49(5):421-429.
9. Moraa I, Sturman N, McGuire T, van Driel ML. Heliox for croup in children. *Cochrane Database Syst Rev.* 7 December 2013;(12):CD006822.
10. Thompson M, Vodicka TA, Blair PS, et al. Duration of symptoms of respiratory tract infections in children: systematic review. TARGET Programme Team. *BMJ.* 2013;347:f7027.
11. Dobrovoljac M, Geelhoed GC. 27 years of croup: an update highlighting the effectiveness of 0.15 mg/kg of dexamethasone. *Emerg Med Australas.* August 2009;21(4):309-314.

22. C-SPINE INJURY/CLEARANCE

1. Oteir AO, Smith K, Stoelwinder JU, Middleton J, Jennings PA. Should suspected cervical spinal cord injury be immobilised?: a systematic review. *Injury.* April 2015;46(4):528-535.
2. Rhee P, Kuncir EJ, Johnson L, et al. Cervical spine injury is highly dependent on the mechanism of injury following blunt and penetrating assault. *J Traum.* 2006;61(5):1166.
3. Stiell IG, Wells GA, Vandemheen KL, et al. The Canadian C-spine rule for radiography in alert and stable trauma patients. *JAMA.* 17 October 2001;286(15):1841-1848.
4. Greenbaum J, Walters N, Levy PD. An evidenced-based approach to radiographic assessment of cervical spine injuries in the emergency department. *J Emerg Med.* 2009;36(1):64.
5. Kanwar R, Delasobera BE, Hudson K, Frohna W. Emergency department evaluation and treatment of cervical spine injuries. *Emerg Med Clin North Am.* May 2015;33(2):241-282.
6. Hoffman JR, Mower WR, Wolfson AB, Todd KH, Zucker MI. Validity of a set of clinical criteria to rule out injury to the cervical spine in patients with blunt trauma. National Emergency X Radiography Utilization Study Group. *N Engl J Med.* 2000;343(2):94.
7. Garton HJ, Hammer MR. Detection of pediatric cervical spine injury. *Neurosurgery.* March 2008;62(3):700-708.

8. Hoffman JR, Wolfson AB, Todd K, Mower WR. Selective cervical spine radiography in blunt trauma: methodology of the National Emergency X-Radiography Utilization Study (NEXUS). *Ann Emerg Med.* 1998;32(4):461.
9. Griffen MM, Frykberg ER, Kerwin AJ, et al. Radiographic clearance of blunt cervical spine injury: plain radiograph or computed tomography scan? *J Trauma*. August 2003;55(2):222-226.
10. Breslin K, Agrawal D. The use of methylprednisolone in acute spinal cord injury: a review of the evidence, controversies, and recommendations. *Pediatr Emerg Care.* 2012;28(11):1238.

23. CVA

1. Jauch EC, Saver JL, Adams HP Jr, et al. Guidelines for the early management of patients with acute ischemic stroke: a guideline for healthcare professionals from the American Heart Association/American Stroke Association. *Stroke.* 2013;44(3):870.
2. Worster A. ACP Journal Club. Review: 3 prediction rules, particularly ABCD, identify ED patients who can be discharged with low risk for stroke after TIA. *Ann Intern Med.* 15 September 2009;151(6):JC3-JC15.
3. Demaerschalk BM, Kleindorfer DO, Adeoye OM, et al. Scientific rationale for the inclusion and exclusion criteria for intravenous alteplase in acute ischemic stroke: a statement for healthcare professionals from the American Heart Association/American Stroke Association. *Stroke.* 2016;47:581.
4. Summers D, Leonard A, Wentworth D, et al. Comprehensive overview of nursing and interdisciplinary care of the acute ischemic stroke patient: a scientific statement from the American Heart Association. *Stroke.* 2009;40(8):2911.
5. Burns JD, Green DM, Metivier K, DeFusco C. Intensive care management of acute ischemic stroke. *Emerg Med Clin North Am.* 2012;30(3):713.
6. Broderick J, Connolly S, Feldmann E, et al. Guidelines for the management of spontaneous intracerebral hemorrhage in adults: 2007 update: a guideline from the American Heart Association/American Stroke Association Stroke Council, High Blood Pressure Research Council, and the Quality of Care and Outcomes in Research Interdisciplinary Working Group. *Stroke.* 2007;38(6):2001.
7. Xian Y, Holloway RG, Chan PS, et al. Association between stroke center hospitalization for acute ischemic stroke and mortality. *JAMA.* 26 January 2011;305(4):373-380.

24. CYCLIC VOMITING SYNDROME

1. Li BU. Cyclic vomiting syndrome: light emerging from the black box. *J Pediatr.* 1999;135(3):276.
2. Gee S. On fitful or recurrent vomiting. *St Bartholomew Hospital Reports.* 1882;18:1.
3. Li BU, Lefevre F, Chelimsky GG, et al. North American Society for Pediatric Gastroenterology, Hepatology, and Nutrition consensus statement on the diagnosis and management of cyclic vomiting syndrome. *J Pediatr Gastroenterol Nutr.* 2008;47(3):379.

4. Allen JH, de Moore GM, Heddle R, Twartz JC. Cannabinoid hyperemesis: cyclical hyperemesis in association with chronic cannabis abuse. *Gut.* November 2004;53(11):1566-1570.
5. Pareek N, Fleisher DR, Abell T. Cyclic vomiting syndrome: what a gastroenterologist needs to know. *Am J Gastroenterol.* December 2007;102(12):2832-2840.
6. Welch KM. Scientific basis of migraine: speculation on the relationship to cyclic vomiting. *Dig Dis Sci.* 1999;44(8 Suppl):26S.
7. Tan ML, Liwanag MJ, Quak SH. Cyclical vomiting syndrome: recognition, assessment and management. *World J Clin Pediatr.* 8 August 2014;3(3):54-58.
8. Allen JH, de Moore GM, Heddle R, Twartz JC. Cannabinoid hyperemesis: cyclical hyperemesis in association with chronic cannabis abuse. *Gut.* 2004;53(11):1566.
9. Stanghellini V, Chan FK, Hasler WL, et al. Gastroduodenal disorders. *Gastroenterology.* May 2016;150(6):1380-1392.
10. Li BU, Lefevre F, Chelimsky GG, et al. North American Society for Pediatric Gastroenterology, Hepatology, and Nutrition consensus statement on the diagnosis and management of cyclic vomiting syndrome. *J Pediatr Gastroenterol Nutr.* September 2008;47(3):379-393.
11. Boles RG, Chun N, Senadheera D, Wong LJC. Cyclic vomiting syndrome and mitochondrial DNA mutations. *Lancet.* 1997;350(9087):1299.
12. Boles RG, Lovett-Barr MR, Preston A, Li BU, Adams K. Treatment of cyclic vomiting syndrome with co-enzyme Q10 and amitriptyline, a retrospective study. *BMC Neurol* 2010;10:10.
13. Boles RG, Adams K, Ito M, Li BU. Maternal inheritance in cyclic vomiting syndrome with neuromuscular disease. *Am J Med Genet A.* 2003;120A(4):474.
14. Prakash C, Clouse RE. Cyclic vomiting syndrome in adults: clinical features and response to tricyclic antidepressants. *Am J Gastroenterol.* 1999;94(10):2855.
15. Boles RG. High degree of efficacy in the treatment of cyclic vomiting syndrome with combined co-enzyme Q10, L-carnitine and amitriptyline, a case series. *BMC Neurol.* 2011;11:102.
16. Aschenbrenner DS. The FDA limits maximum IV dose of Ondansetron. *Am J Nur.* October 2012;112(10):48.

25. DENTAL ABSCESS

1. Robertson DP, Keys W, Rautemaa-Richardson R, Burns R, Smith AJ. Management of severe acute dental infections. *BMJ.* 24 March 2015;350:h1300.
2. Chow AW. Infections of the oral cavity, neck and head. In: Mandell GL, Dolin R, Blaser MJ, eds. *Principles and practices of infectious diseases.* 8th ed. Philadelphia, PA: Elsevier Churchill Livingstone, 2014:789.
3. Hurley MC, Heran MK. Imaging studies for head and neck infections. *Infect Dis Clin North Am.* 2007;21(2):305.

4. Brook I. Antibiotic resistance of oral anaerobic bacteria and their effect on the management of upper respiratory tract and head and neck infections. *Semin Respir Infect.* 2002;17(3):195.
5. Merry AF, Gibbs RD, Edward J, et al. Combined acetaminophen and ibuprofen for pain relief after oral surgery in adults: a randomized controlled trial. *Br J Anaesth.* January 2010;104(1):80-88.
6. Denisco RC, Kenna GA, O'Neil MG, et al. Prevention of prescription opioid abuse: the role of the dentist. *J Am Dent Assoc.* July 2011;142(7):800-810.
7. Baumgartner JC, Xia T. Antibiotic susceptibility of bacteria associated with endodontic abscesses. *J Endod.* January 2003;29(1):44-47.

26. DIABETIC KETOACIDOSIS

1. Kitabchi AE, Umpierrez GE, Miles JM, Fisher JN. Hyperglycemic crises in adult patients with diabetes. *Diabetes Care.* July 2009;32(7):1335-1343.
2. Fulop M, Tannenbaum H, Dreyer N. Ketotic hyperosmolar coma. *Lancet.* 1973;2(7830):635.
3. Kebler R, McDonald FD, Cadnapaphornchai P. Dynamic changes in serum phosphorus levels in diabetic ketoacidosis. *Am J Med.* 1985;79(5):571.
4. Sheikh-Ali M, Karon BS, Basu A, et al. Can serum beta-hydroxybutyrate be used to diagnose diabetic ketoacidosis? *Diabetes Care.* April 2008;31(4):643-647.
5. Kitabchi AE, Umpierrez GE, Miles JM, Fisher JN. Hyperglycemic crises in adult patients with diabetes. *Diabetes Care.* 2009;32(7):1335.
6. Kitabchi AE, Murphy MB, Spencer J, Matteri R, Karas J. Is a priming dose of insulin necessary in a low-dose insulin protocol for the treatment of diabetic ketoacidosis? *Diabetes Care.* 2008;31(11):2081.
7. Umpierrez GE, Latif K, Stoever J, et al. Efficacy of subcutaneous insulin lispro versus continuous intravenous regular insulin for the treatment of patients with diabetic ketoacidosis. *Am J Med.* 2004;117(5):291.
8. Umpierrez GE, Cuervo R, Karabell A, Latif K, Freire AX, Kitabchi AE. Treatment of diabetic ketoacidosis with subcutaneous insulin aspart. *Diabetes Care.* 2004;27(8):1873.
9. Beigelman PM. Potassium in severe diabetic ketoacidosis. *Am J Med.* 1973;54(4):419.
10. Upala S, Jaruvongvanich V, Wijarnpreecha K. Hypomagnesemia and mortality in patients admitted to intensive care unit: a systematic review and meta-analysis. *QJM.* July 2016;109(7):453-459.
11. Wolfsdorf J, Glaser N, Sperling MA. Diabetic ketoacidosis in infants, children, and adolescents: a consensus statement from the American Diabetes Association. *American Diabetes Association Diabetes Care.* 2006;29(5):1150.
12. Bonkowsky JL, Filloux FM. Extrapontine myelinolysis in a pediatric case of diabetic ketoacidosis and cerebral edema. *J Child Neurol.* February 2003;18(2):144-147.

27. DIVERTICULITIS

1. Sugihara K, Muto T, Morioka Y, Asano A, Yamamoto T. Diverticular disease of the colon in Japan. A review of 615 cases. *Dis Colon Rectum.* 1984;27(8):531.
2. Nagorney DM, Adson MA, Pemberton JH. Sigmoid diverticulitis with perforation and generalized peritonitis. *Dis Colon Rectum.* 1985;28(2):71.
3. Ambrosetti P, Robert JH, Witzig JA, et al. Acute left colonic diverticulitis: a prospective analysis of 226 consecutive cases. *Surgery.* 1994;115(5):546.
4. Wilkins T, Embry K, George R. Diagnosis and management of acute diverticulitis. *Am Fam Physician.* 1 May 2013;87(9):612-620.
5. Laméris W, van Randen A, Bipat S, et al. Graded compression ultrasonography and computed tomography in acute colonic diverticulitis: meta-analysis of test accuracy. *Eur Radiol.* November 2008;18(11):2498-2511.
6. Biondo S, Golda T, Kreisler E, et al. Outpatient versus hospitalization management for uncomplicated diverticulitis: a prospective, multicenter randomized clinical trial (DIVER Trial). *Ann Surg.* 2014;259(1):38.
7. Feingold D, Steele SR, Lee S, et al. Practice parameters for the treatment of sigmoid diverticulitis. *Dis Colon Rectum.* March 2014;57(3):284-294.
8. Schechter S, Mulvey J, Eisenstat TE. Management of uncomplicated acute diverticulitis: results of a survey. *Dis Colon Rectum.* 1999;42(4):470.
9. Lau KC, Spilsbury K, Farooque Y, et al. Is colonoscopy still mandatory after a CT diagnosis of left-sided diverticulitis: can colorectal cancer be confidently excluded? *Dis Colon Rectum.* 2011;54(10):1265.

28. EPIGLOTTITIS

1. Rotta AT, Wiryawan B. Respiratory emergencies in children. *Respir Care.* March 2003;48(3):248-258; discussion 258-260.
2. Abdallah C. Acute epiglottitis: trends, diagnosis and management. *Saudi J Anaesth.* July-September 2012;6(3):279-281.
3. Shah RK, Roberson DW, Jones DT. Epiglottitis in the Hemophilus influenzae type B vaccine era: changing trends. *Laryngoscope.* 2004;114(3):557.
4. Mayo-Smith MF, Spinale JW, Donskey CJ, Yukawa M, Li RH, Schiffman FJ. Acute epiglottitis. An 18-year experience in Rhode Island. *Chest.* 1995;108(6):1640.
5. Chroboczek T, Cour M, Hernu R, et al. Long-term outcome of critically ill adult patients with acute epiglottitis. *PLoS One.* 2015;10(5):e0125736.
6. Hammer J. Acquired upper airway obstruction. *Paediatr Respir Rev.* March 2004;5(1):25-33.
7. Ng HL, Sin LM, Li MF, Que TL, Anandaciva S. Acute epiglottitis in adults: a retrospective review of 106 patients in Hong Kong. *Emerg Med J.* 2008;25(5):253.
8. Damm M, Eckel HE, Jungehülsing M, Roth B. Management of acute inflammatory childhood stridor. *Otolaryngol Head Neck Surg.* 1999;121(5):633.

9. Ragosta KG, Orr R, Detweiler MJ. Revisiting epiglottitis: a protocol—the value of lateral neck radiographs. *J Am Osteopath Assoc.* 1997;97(4):227.
10. Schumaker HM, Doris PE, Birnbaum G. Radiographic parameters in adult epiglottitis. *Ann Emerg Med.* 1984;13(8):588.
11. Glynn F, Fenton JE. Diagnosis and management of supraglottitis (epiglottitis). *Curr Infect Dis Rep.* 2008;10(3):200.
12. Sobol SE, Zapata S. Epiglottitis and croup. *Otolaryngol Clin North Am.* 2008;41(3):551.
13. Rotta AT, Wiryawan B. Respiratory emergencies in children. *Respir Care.* March 2003;48(3):248-258; discussion 258-260.
14. Shah RK, Roberson DW, Jones DT. Epiglottitis in the Hemophilus influenzae type B vaccine era: changing trends. *Laryngoscope.* 2004;114(3):557.
15. Zoorob R, Sidani MA, Fremont RD, Kihlberg C. Antibiotic use in acute upper respiratory tract infections. *Am Fam Physician.* 1 November 2012;86(9):817-822.
16. O'Brien WT Sr, Lattin GE Jr. "My airway is closing". *J Fam Pract.* May 2005;54(5):423-425.
17. Baxter FJ, Dunn GL. Acute epiglottitis in adults. *Can J Anaesth.* 1988;35(4):428.
18. Guardiani E, Bliss M, Harley E. Supraglottitis in the era following widespread immunization against Haemophilus influenzae type B: evolving principles in diagnosis and management. *Laryngoscope.* November 2010;120(11):2183-2188.
19. Sack JL, Brock CD. Identifying acute epiglottitis in adults. High degree of awareness, close monitoring are key. *Postgrad Med.* July 2002;112(1):81-82, 85-86.

29. EPISTAXIS

1. Alvi A, Joyner-Triplett N. Acute epistaxis. How to spot the source and stop the flow. *Postgrad Med.* 1996;99(5):83.
2. Petruson B, Rudin R, Svärdsudd K. Is high blood pressure an aetiological factor in epistaxis? *ORL J Otorhinolaryngol Relat Spec.* 1977;39(3):155.
3. Viehweg TL, Roberson JB, Hudson JW. Epistaxis: diagnosis and treatment. *J Oral Maxillofac Surg.* 2006;64(3):511.
4. McGarry GW, Gatehouse S, Hinnie J. Relation between alcohol and nose bleeds. *BMJ.* 1994;309(6955):640.
5. Shakeel M, Trinidade A, Iddamalgoda T, Supriya M, Ah-See KW. Routine clotting screen has no role in the management of epistaxis: reiterating the point. *Eur Arch Otorhinolaryngol.* 2010;267(10):1641.
6. Hodgson D, Burdett-Smith P. Towards evidence-based emergency medicine: best BETs from the Manchester Royal Infirmary. BET 2: routine coagulation testing in adult patients with epistaxis. *Emerg Med J.* July 2011;28(7):633-634.
7. Morgan DJ, Kellerman R. Epistaxis: evaluation and treatment. *Prim Care.* March 2014;41(1):63-73.
8. Krempl GA, Noorily AD. Use of oxymetazoline in the management of epistaxis. *Ann Otol Rhinol Laryngol.* 1995;104(9 Pt 1):704.

9. Middleton PM. Epistaxis. *Emerg Med Australas.* 2004;16(5-6):428.
10. Zahid R, Moharamzadeh P, Alizadeharasi S, Ghasemi A, Saeedi M. A new and rapid method for epistaxis treatment using injectable form of tranexamic acid topically: a randomized controlled trial. *Am J Emerg Med.* September 2013;31(9):1389-1392.
11. Singer AJ, Blanda M, Cronin K, et al. Comparison of nasal tampons for the treatment of epistaxis in the emergency department: a randomized controlled trial. *Ann Emerg Med.* 2005;45(2):134.
12. Pollice PA, Yoder MG. Epistaxis: a retrospective review of hospitalized patients. *Otolaryngol Head Neck Surg.* 1997;117(1):49.

30. ERYTHEMA MULTIFORME

1. Assier H, Bastuji-Garin S, Revuz J, Roujeau JC. Erythema multiforme with mucous membrane involvement and Stevens-Johnson syndrome are clinically different disorders with distinct causes. *Arch Dermatol.* 1995;131(5):539.
2. Sassolas B, Haddad C, Mockenhaupt M, et al. ALDEN, an algorithm for assessment of drug causality in Stevens-Johnson Syndrome and toxic epidermal necrolysis: comparison with case-control analysis. *Clin Pharmacol Ther.* July 2010;88(1):60-68.
3. Huff JC, Weston WL, Tonnesen MG. Erythema multiforme: a critical review of characteristics, diagnostic criteria, and causes. *J Am Acad Dermatol.* 1983;8(6):763.
4. Huff JC. Erythema multiforme. *Dermatol Clin.* 1985;3(1):141.
5. Lamoreux MR, Sternbach MR, Hsu WT. Erythema multiforme. *Am Fam Physician.* 1 December 2006;74(11):1883-1888.
6. Ladizinski B, Carter JB, Lee KC, Aaron DM. Diagnosis of herpes simplex virus-induced erythema multiforme confounded by previous infection with Mycoplasma pneumonia. *J Drugs Dermatol.* 1 June 2013;12(6):707-709.
7. Bean SF, Quezada RK. Recurrent oral erythema multiforme. Clinical experience with 11 patients. *JAMA.* 1983;249(20):2810.
8. Sokumbi O, Wetter DA. Clinical features, diagnosis, and treatment of erythema multiforme: a review for the practicing dermatologist. *Int J Dermatol.* August 2012;51(8):889-902.
9. Creamer D, Walsh SA, Dziewulski P, et al. U.K. guidelines for the management of Stevens-Johnson syndrome/toxic epidermal necrolysis in adults 2016. *Br J Dermatol.* June 2016;174(6):1194-1227.
10. Schwartz RA, McDonough PH, Lee BW. Toxic epidermal necrolysis: Part II. Prognosis, sequelae, diagnosis, differential diagnosis, prevention, and treatment. *J Am Acad Dermatol.* August 2013;69(2):187.e1-187.e16; quiz 203-204.
11. Choonhakarn C, Limpawattana P, Chaowattanapanit S. Clinical profiles and treatment outcomes of systemic corticosteroids for toxic epidermal necrolysis: a retrospective study. *J Dermatol.* February 2016;43(2):156-161.

31. ETHYLENE GLYCOL AND METHANOL TOXICITY

1. Sivilotti ML, Burns MJ, McMartin KE, Brent J. Toxicokinetics of ethylene glycol during fomepizole therapy: implications for management. *Ann Emerg Med.* 2000;36(2):114.
2. Kerns W II, Tomaszewski C, McMartin K, et al. Formate kinetics in methanol poisoning. Methylpyrazole for Toxic Alcohols. *J Toxicol Clin Toxicol.* 2002;40(2):137.
3. Gabow PA, Clay K, Sullivan JB, Lepoff R. Organic acids in ethylene glycol intoxication. *Ann Intern Med.* 1986;105(1):16.
4. Barceloux DG, Krenzelok EP, Olson K, Watson W. American Academy of Clinical Toxicology Practice Guidelines on the Treatment of Ethylene Glycol Poisoning. Ad Hoc Committee. *J Toxicol Clin Toxicol.* 1999;37(5):537.
5. Casavant MJ, Shah MN, Battels R. Does fluorescent urine indicate antifreeze ingestion by children? *Pediatrics.* 2001;107(1):113.
6. Wallace KL, Suchard JR, Curry SC, Reagan C. Diagnostic use of physicians' detection of urine fluorescence in a simulated ingestion of sodium fluorescein-containing antifreeze. *Ann Emerg Med.* 2001;38(1):49.
7. McMartin KE, Sebastian CS, Dies D, Jacobsen D. Kinetics and metabolism of fomepizole in healthy humans. *Clin Toxicol* (Phila). June 2012;50(5):375-383.
8. Nath R, Thind SK, Murthy MS, Farooqui S, Gupta R, Koul HK. Role of pyridoxine in oxalate metabolism. *Ann NY Acad Sci.* 1990;585:274-284.
9. Cheng JT, Beysolow TD, Kaul B, Weisman R, Feinfeld DA. Clearance of ethylene glycol by kidneys and hemodialysis. *J Toxicol Clin Toxicol.* 1987;25(1-2):95-108.

32. FEVER UNKNOWN ORIGIN

1. Petersdorf RG, Beeson PB. Fever of unexplained origin: report on 100 cases. *Medicine* (Baltimore). 1961;40:1.
2. Hayakawa K, Ramasamy B, Chandrasekar PH. Fever of unknown origin: an evidence-based review. *Am J Med Sci.* October 2012;344(4):307-316.
3. Hersch EC, Oh RC. Prolonged febrile illness and fever of unknown origin in adults. *Am Fam Physician.* 15 July 2014;90(2):91-96.
4. Freifeld AG, Bow EJ, Sepkowitz KA, et al. Clinical practice guideline for the use of antimicrobial agents in neutropenic patients with cancer: 2010 update by the infectious diseases society of America. *Clin Infect Dis.* 15 February 2011;52(4):e56-e93.

33. FIFTH DISEASE

1. Anderson LJ. Role of parvovirus B19 in human disease. *Pediatr Infect Dis J.* 1987; 6(8):711.
2. Waldman M, Kopp JB. Parvovirus B19 and the kidney. *Clin J Am Soc Nephrol.* 2007;2 Suppl 1:S47.

3. Servey JT, Reamy BV, Hodge J. Clinical presentations of parvovirus B19 infection. *Am Fam Physician.* 1 February 2007;75(3):373-376.
4. Mandel ED. Erythema infectiosum: recognizing the many faces of fifth disease. *JAAPA.* June 2009;22(6):42-46.

34. FOREIGN BODIES

1. Halaas GW. Management of foreign bodies in the skin. *Am Fam Physician.* 1 September 2007;76(5):683-688.
2. Wyllie R. Foreign bodies in the gastrointestinal tract. *Curr Opin Pediatr.* 2006;18(5):563.
3. Uyemura MC. Foreign body ingestion in children. *Am Fam Physician.* 2005;72(2):287.
4. Schlesinger AE, Crowe JE. Sagittal orientation of ingested coins in the esophagus in children. *AJR Am J Roentgenol.* 2011;196(3):670.
5. Hussain SZ, Bousvaros A, Gilger M, et al. Management of ingested magnets in children. *J Pediatr Gastroenterol Nutr.* September 2012;55(3);239-242.
6. Litovitz T, Whitaker N, Clark L, White NC, Marsolek M. Emerging battery-ingestion hazard: clinical implications. *Pediatrics.* 2010;125(6):1168.

35. GI BLEED

1. Srygley FD, Gerardo CJ, Tran T, Fisher DA. Does this patient have a severe upper gastrointestinal bleed? *JAMA.* 14 March 2012;307(10):1072-1079.
2. Wilkins T, Khan N, Nabh A, Schade RR. Diagnosis and management of upper gastrointestinal bleeding. *Am Fam Physician.* 1 March 2012;85(5):469-476.
3. Barkun A, Bardou M, Marshall JK, Nonvariceal Upper GI Bleeding Consensus Conference Group. Consensus recommendations for managing patients with nonvariceal upper gastrointestinal bleeding. *Ann Intern Med.* 2003;139(10):843.
4. Laine L, Jensen D. Management of patients with ulcer bleeding. *Am J Gastroenterol.* March 2012;107:345-360.
5. Cappell MS, Friedel D. Initial management of acute upper gastrointestinal bleeding: from initial evaluation up to gastrointestinal endoscopy. *Med Clin North Am.* 2008;92(3):491.
6. Ryan ML, Thorson CM, Otero CA, et al. Initial hematocrit in trauma: a paradigm shift? *J Trauma Acute Care Surg.* January 2012;72(1):54-59.
7. Bruns B, Lindsey M, Rowe K, et al. Hemoglobin drops within minutes of injuries and predicts need for an intervention to stop hemorrhage. *J Trauma.* August 2007;63(2):312-315.
8. Pallin DJ, Saltzman JR. Is nasogastric tube lavage in patients with acute upper GI bleeding indicated or antiquated? *Gastrointest Endosc.* 2011;74(5):981.
9. Baradarian R, Ramdhaney S, Chapalamadugu R, et al. Early intensive resuscitation of patients with upper gastrointestinal bleeding decreases mortality. *Am J Gastroenterol.* 2004;99(4):619.

10. Villanueva C, Colomo A, Bosch A, et al. Transfusion strategies for acute upper gastrointestinal bleeding. *N Engl J Med.* 2013;368(1):11.
11. Green FW Jr, Kaplan MM, Curtis LE, Levine PH. Effect of acid and pepsin on blood coagulation and platelet aggregation. A possible contributor prolonged gastroduodenal mucosal hemorrhage. *Gastroenterology.* 1978;74(1):38.
12. Bennett C, Klingenberg SL, Langholz E, Gluud LL. Tranexamic acid for upper gastrointestinal bleeding. *Cochrane Database Syst Rev.* 21 November 2014;(11):CD006640.
13. Blatchford O, Murray WR, Blatchford M. A risk score to predict need for treatment for upper-gastrointestinal haemorrhage. *Lancet.* 2000;356(9238):1318.
14. Le Jeune IR, Gordon AL, Farrugia D, Manwani R, Guha IN, James MW. Safe discharge of patients with low-risk upper gastrointestinal bleeding (UGIB): can the use of Glasgow-Blatchford Bleeding Score be extended? *Acute Med.* 2011;10(4):176-181.
15. Gralnek IM. Outpatient management of "low-risk" nonvariceal upper GI hemorrhage. Are we ready to put evidence into practice? *Gastrointest Endosc.* January 2002;55(1):131-134.

36. GLAUCOMA

1. Prum BE Jr, Rosenberg LF, Gedde SJ, et al. Primary open-angle glaucoma preferred practice pattern guidelines. *Ophthalmology.* 2016;123(1):41.
2. Kingman S. Glaucoma is the second leading cause of blindness globally. *Bull World Health Organ.* 2004;82(11):887.
3. Quigley HA. Glaucoma. *Lancet.* 16 April 2011;377(9774):1367-1377.
4. Worley A, Grimmer-Somers K. Risk factors for glaucoma: what do they really mean? *Aust J Prim Health.* 2011;17(3):233-239.
5. Leibowitz HM. The red eye. *N Engl J Med.* 2000;343(5):345.
6. Fresco BB. A new tonometer—the pressure phosphene tonometer: clinical comparison with Goldman tonometry. *Ophthalmology.* November 1998;105(11):2123-2126.
7. Tanna AP, Budenz DL, Bandi J, et al. Glaucoma progression analysis software compared with expert consensus opinion in the detection of visual field progression in glaucoma. *Ophthalmology.* March 2012;119(3):468-473.
8. Bonomi L, Marchini G, Marraffa M, Morbio R. The relationship between intraocular pressure and glaucoma in a defined population. Data from the Egna–Neumarkt glaucoma study. *Ophthalmologica.* January-February 2001;215(1):34-38.
9. Mohammadi SF, Mirhadi S, Mehrjardi HZ, et al. An algorithm for glaucoma screening in clinical settings and its preliminary performance profile. *J Ophthalmic Vis Res.* October 2013;8(4):314-320.
10. Aung T, Ang LP, Chan SP, Chew PT. Acute primary angle-closure: long-term intraocular pressure outcome in Asian eyes. *Am J Ophthalmol.* January 2001;131(1):7-12.
11. Shields SR. Managing eye disease in primary care. Part 3. When to refer for ophthalmologic care. *Postgrad Med.* 2000;108(5):99.

12. American Optometric Association. *Optometric Clinical Practice Guideline: Care of the Patient With Primary Angle Closure Glaucoma.* St. Louis, MO: American Optometric Association, 1994.

37. HEADACHE

1. Cady RK, Schreiber CP. Sinus headache or migraine? Considerations in making a differential diagnosis. *Neurology.* 2002;58(9 Suppl 6):S10.
2. Lipton RB, Bigal ME, Steiner TJ, Silberstein SD, Olesen J. Classification of primary headaches. *Neurology.* 2004;63(3):427.
3. Hainer BL, Matheson EM. Approach to acute headache in adults. *Am Fam Physician.* 15 May 2013;87(10):682-687.
4. Buring JE, Hebert P, Romero J, et al. Migraine and subsequent risk of stroke in the Physicians' Health Study. *Arch Neurol.* 1995;52(2):129.
5. Hagen K, Stovner LJ, Vatten L, Holmen J, Zwart JA, Bovim G. Blood pressure and risk of headache: a prospective study of 22,685 adults in Norway. *J Neurol Neurosurg Psychiatry.* 2002;72(4):463.
6. Gil-Gouveia R, Martins IP. Headaches associated with refractive errors: myth or reality? *Headache.* 2002;42(4):256.
7. Walker HK, Hall WD, Hurst JW, eds. *Clinical Methods: The History, Physical, and Laboratory Examinations.* 3rd ed. Boston, MA: Butterworths, 1990.
8. Tsushima Y, Endo K. MR imaging in the evaluation of chronic or recurrent headache. *Radiology.* 2005;235(2):575.
9. Perry JJ, Stiell IG, Sivilotti ML, et al. Clinical decision rules to rule out subarachnoid hemorrhage for acute headache. *JAMA.* 25 September 2013;310(12):1248-1255.
10. Edlow JA, Caplan LR. Avoiding pitfalls in the diagnosis of subarachnoid hemorrhage. *N Engl J Med.* 2000;342(1):29.
11. Douglas AC, Wippold FJ 2nd, Broderick DF, et al. ACR Appropriateness Criteria Headache. *J Am Coll Radiol.* July 2014;11(7):657-667.
12. Gonzalez-Gay MA, Lopez-Diaz MJ, Barros S, et al. Giant cell arteritis: laboratory tests at the time of diagnosis in a series of 240 patients. *Medicine* (Baltimore). September 2005;84(5):277-290.
13. Evans RW. Diagnostic testing for the evaluation of headaches. *Neurol Clin.* February 1996;14(1):1-26.
14. Evers S, Goadsby P, Jensen R, May A, Pascual J, Sixt G. Treatment of miscellaneous idiopathic headache disorders (Group 4 of the IHS classification)—report of an EFNS task force. *Eur J Neurol.* June 2011;18(6):803-812.

38. HEART FAILURE

1. Watson RDS, Gibbs CR, Lip GYH. ABC of heart failure: clinical features and complications. *BMJ.* 22 January 2000;320(7229): 236-239.

2. Allen LA, O'Connor CM. Management of acute decompensated heart failure. *CMAJ*. 13 March 2007;176(6):797-805.
3. Dosh SA. Diagnosis of heart failure in adults. *Am Fam Physician*. 1 December 2004;70(11):2145-2152.
4. Park JH, Balmain S, Berry C, Morton JJ, McMurray JJ. Potentially detrimental cardiovascular effects of oxygen in patients with chronic left ventricular systolic dysfunction. *Heart*. April 2010;96(7):533-538.
5. Yancy CW, Jessup M, Bozkurt B, et al. 2013 ACCF/AHA guideline for the management of heart failure: a report of the American College of Cardiology Foundation/American Heart Association Task Force on practice guidelines. *Circ*. 15 October 2013;128(16):e240-e327.
6. Elkayam U, Bitar F, Akhter MW, Khan S, Patrus S, Derakhshani M. Intravenous nitroglycerin in the treatment of decompensated heart failure: potential benefits and limitations. *J Cardiovasc Pharmacol Ther*. December 2004;9(4):227-241.
7. Mullens W, Abrahams Z, Francis GS, et al. Sodium nitroprusside for advanced low-output heart failure. *J Am Coll Cardiol*. 15 July 2008;52(3):200-207.
8. Graff L, Orledge J, Radford MJ, Wang Y, Petrillo M, Maag R. Correlation of the Agency for Health Care Policy and Research congestive heart failure admission guideline with mortality: peer review organization voluntary hospital association initiative to decrease events (PROVIDE) for congestive heart failure. *Ann Emerg Med*. October 1999;34(4 Pt 1):429-437.

39. HEMOPTYSIS

1. Corder R. Hemoptysis. *Emerg Med Clin North Am*. May 2003;21(2):421-435.
2. Poe RH, Israel RH, Marin MG, et al. Utility of fiberoptic bronchoscopy in patients with hemoptysis and a nonlocalizing chest roentgenogram. *Chest*. 1988;93(1):70.
3. Ketai LH, Mohammed TL, Kirsch J, et al. ACR appropriateness criteria® hemoptysis. *J Thorac Imaging*. 2014;29(3):19.
4. Revel MP, Fournier LS, Hennebicque AS, et al. Can CT replace bronchoscopy in the detection of the site and cause of bleeding in patients with large or massive hemoptysis? *AJR Am J Roentgenol*. 2002;179(5):1217.
5. Larici AR, Franchi P, Occhipinti M, et al. Diagnosis and management of hemoptysis. *Diagn Interv Radiol*. July-August 2014;20(4):299-309.
6. Earwood JS, Thompson TD. Hemoptysis: evaluation and management. *Am Fam Physician*. 15 February 2015;91(4):243-249.
7. Khalil A, Soussan M, Mangiapan G, Fartoukh M, Parrot A, Carette MF. Utility of high-resolution chest CT scan in the emergency management of haemoptysis in the intensive care unit: severity, localization and aetiology. *Br J Radiol*. 2007;80(949):21.

40. HERPES ZOSTER

1. Dworkin RH, Johnson RW, Breuer J, et al. Recommendations for the management of herpes zoster. *Clin Infect Dis*. 2007;(44 Suppl 1):S1.

2. Yawn BP, Saddier P, Wollan PC, St Sauver JL, Kurland MJ, Sy LS. A population-based study of the incidence and complication rates of herpes zoster before zoster vaccine introduction. *Mayo Clin Proc.* 2007;82(11):1341.
3. Jumaan AO, Yu O, Jackson LA, Bohlke K, Galil K, Seward JF. Incidence of herpes zoster, before and after varicella-vaccination-associated decreases in the incidence of varicella, 1992-2002. *J Infect Dis.* 2005;191(12):2002.
4. Harger JH, Ernest JM, Thurnau GR, et al. Risk factors and outcome of varicella-zoster virus pneumonia in pregnant women. *J Infect Dis.* 2002;185(4):422.
5. Paryani SG, Arvin AM. Intrauterine infection with varicella-zoster virus after maternal varicella. *N Engl J Med.* 1986;314(24):1542.
6. Hirschmann JV. Herpes zoster. *N Engl J Med.* 31 October 2013;369(18):1765.
7. Dworkin RH, Johnson RW, Breuer J, et al. Recommendations for the management of herpes zoster. *Clin Infect Dis.* 1 January 2007;44 Suppl 1:S1-S26.
8. Adour KK. Otological complications of herpes zoster. *Ann Neurol.* 1994;35 Suppl:S62.
9. Uscategui T, Dorée C, Chamberlain IJ, Burton MJ. Antiviral therapy for Ramsay Hunt syndrome (herpes zoster oticus with facial palsy) in adults. *Cochrane Database Syst Rev.* 8 October 2008;(4):CD006851.
10. Whitley RJ, Weiss H, Gnann JW Jr, et al. Acyclovir with and without prednisone for the treatment of herpes zoster. A randomized, placebo-controlled trial. The National Institute of Allergy and Infectious Diseases Collaborative Antiviral Study Group. *Ann Intern Med.* 1 September 1996;125(5):376-383.
11. Wilson JF. In the clinic. Herpes zoster. *Ann Intern Med.* 1 March 2011;154(5):ITC31-15; quiz ITC316.
12. Hempenstall K, Nurmikko TJ, Johnson RW, A'Hern RP, Rice ASC. Analgesic therapy in postherpetic neuralgia: a quantitative systematic review. *PLoS Med.* 2005; 2(7):e164.
13. Finnerup NB, Attal N, Haroutounian S, et al. Pharmacotherapy for neuropathic pain in adults: a systematic review and meta-analysis. *Lancet Neurol.* 2015;14(2):162.

41. HICCUPS

1. Kolodzik PW, Eilers MA. Hiccups (singultus): review and approach to management. *Ann Emerg Med.* 1991;20(5):565.
2. Samuels L. Hiccup: a ten year review of anatomy, etiology, and treatment. *Can Med Assoc J.* 1952;67(4):315.
3. Calsina-Berna A, García-Gómez G, González-Barboteo J, Porta-Sales J. Treatment of chronic hiccups in cancer patients: a systematic review. *J Palliat Med.* October 2012;15(10):1142-1150.
4. Marinella MA. Diagnosis and management of hiccups in the patient with advanced cancer. *J Support Oncol.* July-August 2009;7(4):122-127; 130.
5. Rousseau P. Hiccups. *South Med J.* 1995;88(2):175.

6. Marsot-Dupuch K, Bousson V, Cabane J, Tubiana JM. Intractable hiccups: the role of cerebral MR in cases without systemic cause. *Am J Neuroradiol.* 1995;16(10):2093.
7. Moretto EN, Wee B, Wiffen PJ, Murchison AG. Interventions for treating persistent and intractable hiccups in adults. *Cochrane Database Syst Rev.* 31 January 2013;(1):CD008768.
8. Peleg R, Peleg A. Case report: sexual intercourse as potential treatment for intractable hiccups. *Can Fam Physician.* August 2000;46:1631-1632.
9. Friedggod CE, Ripstein CB. Chlorpromazine (thorazine) in the treatment of intractable hiccups. *J Am Med Assoc.* 22 Januray 1955;157(4):309-310.
10. Guelaud C, Similowski T, Bizec JL, Cabane J, Whitelaw WA, Derenne JP. Baclofen therapy for chronic hiccup. *Eur Respir J.* February 1995;8(2):235-237.
11. Ramírez FC, Graham DY. Treatment of intractable hiccup with baclofen: results of a double-blind randomized, controlled, cross-over study. *Am J Gastroenterol.* 1992;87(12):1789.
12. Wang T, Wang D. Metoclopramide for patients with intractable hiccups: a multicentre, randomised, controlled pilot study. *Intern Med J.* 2014;44(12a):1205.
13. Porzio G, Aielli F, Verna L, Aloisi P, Galletti B, Ficorella C. Gabapentin in the treatment of hiccups in patients with advanced cancer: a 5-year experience. *Clin Neuropharmacol.* July 2010;33(4):179-180.
14. Kang JH, Bruera E. Hiccups during chemotherapy: what should we do? *J Palliat Med.* 18 July 2015;18(7):572.

42. HIP FRACTURE

1. Brunner LC, Eshilian-Oates L, Kuo TY. Hip fractures in adults. *Am Fam Physician.* 1 February 2003;67(3):537-542.
2. Albertsson DM, Mellström D, Petersson C, Eggertsen R. Validation of a 4-item score predicting hip fracture and mortality risk among elderly women. *Ann Fam Med.* January-February 2007;5(1):48-56.
3. O'Connor PJ. A painful hip. *BMJ.* 15 September 2007;335(7619):563-564.
4. Frihagen F, Nordsletten L, Tariq R, Madsen JE. MRI diagnosis of occult hip fractures. *Acta Orthop.* 2005;76(4):524.
5. Adunsky A, Lichtenstein A, Mizrahi E, Arad M, Heim M. Blood transfusion requirements in elderly hip fracture patients. *Arch Gerontol Geriatr.* 2003;36(1):75.
6. Titler MG, Herr K, Schilling ML, et al. Acute pain treatment for older adults hospitalized with hip fracture: current nursing practices and perceived barriers. *Appl Nurs Res.* 2003;16(4):211.
7. Handoll HH, Queally JM, Parker MJ. Pre-operative traction for hip fractures in adults. *Cochrane Database Syst Rev.* 7 December 2011;(12):CD000168.
8. Moja L, Piatti A, Pecoraro V, et al. Timing matters in hip fracture surgery: patients operated within 48 hours have better outcomes. A meta-analysis and meta-regression of over 190,000 patients. *PLoS One.* 2012;7(10):e46175.

43. HYPERKALEMIA

1. McMorran S. Treatment of hyperkalaemia in the emergency department. *Emerg Med J.* May 2001;18(3):233.
2. Hollander-Rodriguez JC, Calvert JF Jr. Hyperkalemia. *Am Fam Physician.* 15 January 2006;73(2):283-290.
3. Van Mieghem C, Sabbe M, Knockaert D. The clinical value of the ECG in noncardiac conditions. *Chest.* April 2004;125(4):1561-1576.
4. Xu B, Murray M. Persistent hyperkalaemia. *Aust Fam Physician.* May 2009;38(5): 307-309.
5. Debono M; Ross RJ. Doses and steroids to be used in primary and central hypoadrenalism. *Ann Endocrinol* (Paris). 2007;68(4):265-267.
6. Parham WA, Mehdirad AA, Biermann KM, Fredman CS. Hyperkalemia revisited. *Tex Heart Inst J.* 2006;33(1):40-47.
7. Mahoney BA, Smith WA, Lo DS, Tsoi K, Tonelli M, Clase CM. Emergency interventions for hyperkalaemia. *Cochrane Database Syst Rev.* 18 April 2005;(2):CD003235.
8. Varriale P, Ngai L. Sodium polystyrene sulfonate use revisited. *Am J Med.* August 2014;127(8):e37.
9. Sterns RH, Rojas M, Bernstein P, Chennupati S. Ion-exchange resins for the treatment of hyperkalemia: are they safe and effective? *J Am Soc Nephrol.* 2010;21(5):733.
10. Blumberg A, Weidmann P, Shaw S, Gnädinger M. Effect of various therapeutic approaches on plasma potassium and major regulating factors in terminal renal failure. *Am J Med.* 1988;85(4):507.
11. Ingelfinger JR. A new era for the treatment of hyperkalemia? *N Engl J Med.* 2015;372(3):275.
12. Charytan D, Goldfarb DS. Indications for hospitalization of patients with hyperkalemia. *Arch Intern Med.* 2000;160(11):1605-1611.

44. HYPERTENSIVE EMERGENCY

1. U.S. Department of Health and Human Services. *The seventh report of the Joint National Committee on prevention, detection, evaluation, and treatment of high blood pressure* [Internet]. National Heart, Lung, and Blood Institute; [May 2004; cited 18 June 2017]. https://www.nhlbi.nih.gov/files/docs/guidelines/jnc7full.pdf.
2. Katz JN, Gore JM, Amin A, et al. Practice patterns, outcomes, and end-organ dysfunction for patients with acute severe hypertension: the Studying the Treatment of Acute hypertension (STAT) registry. *Am Heart J.* October 2009;158(4):599-606.
3. Zeller KR, Von Kuhnert L, Matthews C. Rapid reduction of severe asymptomatic hypertension. A prospective, controlled trial. *Arch Intern Med.*1989;149(10):2186.
4. Mayer SA, Kurtz P, Wyman A, et al. Clinical practices, complications, and mortality in neurological patients with acute severe hypertension: the studying the treatment of acute hypertension registry. *Crit Care Med.* October 2011;39(10):2330-2336.

5. James PA, Oparil S, Carter BL, et al. 2014 evidence-based guideline for the management of high blood pressure in adults: report from the panel members appointed to the Eighth Joint National Committee (JNC 8). *JAMA*. 5 February 2014;311(5):507-520.
6. Martin JF, Higashiama E, Garcia E, et al. Hypertensive crisis profile. Prevalence and clinical presentation. *Arq Bras Cardiol*. August 2004;83(2):125-130; 131-136.
7. Johnson W, Nguyen ML, Patel R. Hypertension crisis in the emergency department.*Cardiol Cli*. November 2012;30(4):533-543.
8. Varon J, Marik PE. Clinical review: the management of hypertensive crises. *Crit Care*. October 2003;7(5):374-384.
9. Perez MI, Musini VM. Pharmacological interventions for hypertensive emergencies. *Cochrane Database Syst Rev*. 23 January 2008;(1):CD003653.
10. Marik PE, Varon J. Hypertensive crises: challenges and management. *Chest*. June 2007;131(6):1949-1962.
11. Souza LM, Riera R, Saconato H, Demathé A, Atallah AN. Oral drugs for hypertensive urgencies: systematic review and meta-analysis. *Sao Paulo Med J*. November 2009;127(6):366-372.
12. Elliott WJ. Hypertensive emergencies. *Crit Care Clin*. 2001;17(2):435.
13. Papadopoulos DP, Sanidas EA, Viniou NA, Chantziara V, Barbetseas I, Makris TK. Cardiovascular hypertensive emergencies. *Curr Hypertens Rep*. February 2015; 17(2):5.
14. Hemphill JC III, Greenberg SM, Anderson CS, et al. Guidelines for the management of spontaneous intracerebral hemorrhage: a guideline for healthcare professionals from the American Heart Association/American Stroke Association. *Stroke*. July 2015;46(7):2032-2060.
15. Manning L, Robinson TG, Anderson CS. Control of blood pressure in hypertensive neurological emergencies. *Curr Hypertens Rep*. June 2014;16(6):436.

45. HYPOKALEMIA

1. Gennari FJ. Hypokalemia. *N Engl J Med*. 13 August 1998;339(7):451-458.
2. Oram RA, McDonald TJ, Vaidya B. Investigating hypokalaemia. *BMJ*. 24 September 2013;347:f5137.
3. Comi G, Testa D, Cornelio F, Comola M, Canal N. Potassium depletion myopathy: a clinical and morphological study of six cases. *Muscle Nerve*. 1985;8(1):17.
4. Dalal BI, Brigden ML. Factitious biochemical measurements resulting from hematologic conditions. *Am J Clin Pathol*. February 2009;131(2):195-204.
5. Kraft MD, Btaiche IF, Sacks GS, Kudsk KA. Treatment of electrolyte disorders in adult patients in the intensive care unit. *Am J Health Syst Pharm*. 15 August 2005;62(16):1663-1682.
6. Adrogué HJ, Lederer ED, Suki WN, Eknoyan G. Determinants of plasma potassium levels in diabetic ketoacidosis. *Medicine* (Baltimore). 1986;65(3):163.

7. Hamill RJ, Robinson LM, Wexler HR, Moote C. Efficacy and safety of potassium infusion therapy in hypokalemic critically ill patients. *Crit Care Med.* 1991;19(5):694.
8. Drew BJ, Califf RM, Funk M, et al. Practice standards for electrocardiographic monitoring in hospital settings: an American Heart Association scientific statement from the Councils on Cardiovascular Nursing, Clinical Cardiology, and Cardiovascular Disease in the Young: endorsed by the International Society of Computerized Electrocardiology and the American Association of Critical-Care Nurses. *Circulation.* 2004;110(17):2721.
9. Gennari FJ. Hypokalemia. *N Engl J Med.* 1998;339(7):451.
10. Villamil MF, Deland EC, Henney RP, Maloney JV Jr. Anion effects on cation movements during correction of potassium depletion. *Am J Physiol.* 1975;229(1):161.

46. IMPETIGO

1. Bowen AC, Mahé A, Hay RJ, et al. The global epidemiology of impetigo: a systematic review of the population prevalence of impetigo and pyoderma. *PLoS One.* 2015;10(8):e0136789.
2. Dajani AS, Ferrieri P, Wannamaker LW. Natural history of impetigo. II. Etiologic agents and bacterial interactions. *J Clin Invest.* 1972;51(11):2863.
3. Cole C, Gazewood J. Diagnosis and treatment of impetigo. *Am Fam Physician.* 15 May 2007;75(6):859-864.
4. Stevens DL, Bisno AL, Chambers HF, et al. Practice guidelines for the diagnosis and management of skin and soft tissue infections: 2014 update by the infectious diseases society of America. *Clin Infect Dis.* 2014;59(2):147.
5. Siegel JD, Rhinehart E, Jackson M, Chiarello L; Health Care Infection Control Practices Advisory Committee. *2007 Guideline for isolation precautions: preventing transmission of infectious agents in healthcare settings.* [Internet]. Centers for Disease Control and Prevention; [2007; cited 25 May 2017]. https://www.cdc.gov/niosh/docket/archive/pdfs/NIOSH-219/0219-010107-siegel.pdf.
6. Shope TR, Hashikawa AN. Exclusion of mildly ill children from childcare. *Pediatr Ann.* May 2012;41(5):204-208.

47. INFLAMMATORY BOWEL DISEASE

1. Silverberg MS, Satsangi J, Ahmad T, et al. Toward an integrated clinical, molecular and serological classification of inflammatory bowel disease: report of a Working Party of the 2005 Montreal World Congress of Gastroenterology. *Can J Gastroenterol.* 2005;(19 Suppl) A:5A.
2. Grucela A, Steinhagen RM. Current surgical management of ulcerative colitis. *Mt Sinai J Med.* December 2009;76(6):606-612.
3. Feuerstein JD, Cheifetz AS. Ulcerative colitis: epidemiology, diagnosis, and management. *Mayo Clin Proc.* November 2014;89(11):1553-1563.

4. Kornbluth A, Sachar DB. Ulcerative colitis practice guidelines in adults: American College of Gastroenterology, Practice Parameters Committee. *Am J Gastroenterol.* March 2010;105(3):501-523.
5. Poullis AP, Zar S, Sundaram KK, et al. A new, highly sensitive assay for c-reactive protein can aid the differentiation of inflammatory bowel disorders from constipation- and diarrhoea-predominant functional bowel disorders. *Eur J Gastroenterol Hepatol.* 2002;14(4):409.
6. Horsthuis K, Bipat S, Bennink RJ, Stoker J. Inflammatory bowel disease diagnosed with US, MR, scintigraphy, and CT: meta-analysis of prospective studies. *Radiology.* April 2008;247(1):64-79.
7. Biddle WL, Greenberger NJ, Swan JT, McPhee MS, Miner PB Jr. 5-Aminosalicylic acid enemas: effective agent in maintaining remission in left-sided ulcerative colitis. *Gastroenterology.* 1988;94(4):1075.
8. Marteau P, Probert CS, Lindgren S, et al. Combined oral and enema treatment with Pentasa (mesalazine) is superior to oral therapy alone in patients with extensive mild/moderate active ulcerative colitis: a randomised, double blind, placebo controlled study. *Gut.* 2005;54(7):960.
9. Safdi M, DeMicco M, Sninsky C, et al. A double-blind comparison of oral versus rectal mesalamine versus combination therapy in the treatment of distal ulcerative colitis. *Am J Gastroenterol.* 1997;92(10):1867.
10. Nugent FW, Roy MA. Duodenal Crohn's disease: an analysis of 89 cases. *Am J Gastroenterol.* 1989;84(3):249.
11. Steinhart AH, Feagan BG, Wong CJ, et al. Combined budesonide and antibiotic therapy for active Crohn's disease: a randomized controlled trial. *Gastroenterology.* 2002;123(1):33.

48. INTUSSUSCEPTION

1. Waseem M, Rosenberg HK. Intussusception. *Pediatr Emerg Care.* November 2008;24(11):793-800.
2. Erkan N, Haciyanli M, Yildirim M, Sayhan H, Vardar E, Polat AF. Intussusception in adults: an unusual and challenging condition for surgeons. *Int J Colorectal Dis.* 2005;20(5):452.
3. Mandeville K, Chien M, Willyerd FA, Mandell G, Hostetler MA, Bulloch B. Intussusception: clinical presentations and imaging characteristics. *Pediatr Emerg Care.* September 2012;28(9):842-844.
4. West KW, Stephens B, Vane DW, Grosfeld JL. Intussusception: current management in infants and children. *Surgery.* 1987;102(4):704.
5. Tenenbein M, Wiseman NE. Early coma in intussusception: endogenous opioid induced? *Pediatr Emerg Care.* March 1987;3(1):22-23.
6. Losek JD, Fiete RL. Intussusception and the diagnostic value of testing stool for occult blood. *Am J Emerg Med.* 1991;9(1):1.

7. Ko HS, Schenk JP, Tröger J, Rohrschneider WK. Current radiological management of intussusception in children. *Eur Radiol.* 2007;17(9):2411.
8. Saverino BP, Lava C, Lowe LH, Rivard DC. Radiographic findings in the diagnosis of pediatric ileocolic intussusception: comparison to a control population. *Pediatr Emerg Care.* 2010;26(4):281.
9. Navarro O, Daneman A. Intussusception. Part 3: diagnosis and management of those with an identifiable or predisposing cause and those that reduce spontaneously. *Pediatr Radiol.* 2004;34(4):305.
10. Riera A, Hsiao AL, Langhan ML, Goodman TR, Chen L. Diagnosis of intussusception by physician novice sonographers in the emergency department. *Ann Emerg Med.* September 2012;60(3):264-268.
11. Meier DE, Coln CD, Rescorla FJ, OlaOlorun A, Tarpley JL. Intussusception in children: international perspective. *World J Surg.* 1996;20(8):1035.

49. KAWASAKI DISEASE

1. Saguil A, Fargo M, Grogan S. Diagnosis and management of kawasaki disease. *Am Fam Physician.* 15 March 2015;91(6):365-371.
2. Ozdemir H, Ciftçi E, Tapisiz A, et al. Clinical and epidemiological characteristics of children with Kawasaki disease in Turkey. *J Trop Pediatr.* 2010;56(4):260.
3. Burns JC, Glodé MP. Kawasaki syndrome. *Lancet.* 2004;364(9433):533.
4. Shike H, Kanegaye JT, Best BM, Pancheri J, Burns JC. Pyuria associated with acute Kawasaki disease and fever from other causes. *Pediatr Infect Dis J.* 2009;28(5):440.
5. Harnden A, Takahashi M, Burgner D. Kawasaki disease. *BMJ.* 5 May 2009;338:b1514.
6. Newburger JW, Takahashi M, Gerber MA, et al. Diagnosis, treatment, and long-term management of Kawasaki disease: a statement for health professionals from the Committee on Rheumatic Fever, Endocarditis, and Kawasaki Disease, Council on Cardiovascular Disease in the Young, American Heart Association. *Pediatrics.* December 2004;114(6):1708-1733.
7. Yellen ES, Gauvreau K, Takahashi M, et al. Performance of 2004 American Heart Association recommendations for treatment of Kawasaki disease. *Pediatrics.* 2010;125(2):e234.
8. Terai M, Shulman ST. Prevalence of coronary artery abnormalities in Kawasaki disease is highly dependent on gamma globulin dose but independent of salicylate dose. *J Pediatr.* 1997;131(6):888.
9. Giglia TM, Massicotte MP, Tweddell JS, et al. Prevention and treatment of thrombosis in pediatric and congenital heart disease: a scientific statement from the American Heart Association. *Circulation.* 2013;128(24):2622.
10. Terai M, Shulman ST. Prevalence of coronary artery abnormalities in Kawasaki disease is highly dependent on gamma globulin dose but independent of salicylate dose. *J Pediatr.* 1997;131(6):888.

11. Newburger JW, Sleeper LA, McCrindle BW, et al. Randomized trial of pulsed corticosteroid therapy for primary treatment of Kawasaki disease. *N Engl J Med.* 2007;356(7):663.
12. Chen S, Dong Y, Yin Y, Krucoff MW. Intravenous immunoglobulin plus corticosteroid to prevent coronary artery abnormalities in Kawasaki disease: a meta-analysis. *Heart.* January 2013;99(2):76-82.

50. KIDNEY STONE

1. Singh P, Enders FT, Vaughan LE, et al. Stone composition among first-time symptomatic kidney stone formers in the community. *Mayo Clin Proc.* 2015;90(10):1356.
2. Preminger GM, Tiselius HG, Assimos DG, et al. 2007 Guideline for the management of ureteral calculi. *Eur Urol.* December 2007;52(6):1610-1631.
3. Miller OF, Kane CJ Time to stone passage for observed ureteral calculi: a guide for patient education. *J Urol.* September 1999;162(3 Pt 1):688-690; discussion 690-691.
4. Hiatt RA, Ettinger B, Caan B, Quesenberry CP Jr, Duncan D, Citron JT. Randomized controlled trial of a low animal protein, high fiber diet in the prevention of recurrent calcium oxalate kidney stones. *Am J Epidemiol.* 1996;144(1):25.
5. Taylor EN, Fung TT, Curhan GC. DASH-style diet associates with reduced risk for kidney stones. *J Am Soc Nephrol.* 2009;20(10):2253.
6. Press SM, Smith AD. Incidence of negative hematuria in patients with acute urinary lithiasis presenting to the emergency room with flank pain. *Urology.* 1995;45(5):753.
7. Preminger GM, Tiselius HG, Assimos DG, et al. 2007 guideline for the management of ureteral calculi. *J Urol.* 2007;178(6):2418.
8. Pearle MS, Goldfarb DS, Assimos DG, et al. Medical management of kidney stones: AUA guideline. *J Urol.* August 2014;192(2):316-324.
9. Assimos D, Krambeck A, Miller NL, et al. Surgical management of stones: American Urological Association/Endourological Society Guideline, PART II. *J Urol.* October 2016;196(4):1161-1169.
10. Pietrow PK, Karellas ME. Medical management of common urinary calculi. *Am Fam Physician.* 1 July 2006;74(1):86-94.
11. Moore CL, Bomann S, Daniels B, et al. Derivation and validation of a clinical prediction rule for uncomplicated ureteral stone—the STONE score: retrospective and prospective observational cohort studies. *BMJ* . 26 March 2014;348:g2191.
12. Coe FL, Parks JH, Asplin JR. The pathogenesis and treatment of kidney stones. *N Engl J Med.* 1992;327(16):1141.
13. Cordell WH, Wright SW, Wolfson AB, et al. Comparison of intravenous ketorolac, meperidine, and both (balanced analgesia) for renal colic. *Ann Emerg Med.* 1996;28(2):151.
14. Teichman JM. Clinical practice. Acute renal colic from ureteral calculus. *N Engl J Med.* 2004;350(7):684.

15. Safdar B, Degutis LC, Landry K, Vedere SR, Moscovitz HC, D'Onofrio G. Intravenous morphine plus ketorolac is superior to either drug alone for treatment of acute renal colic. *Ann Emerg Med.* 2006;48(2):173.
16. Pickard R, Starr K, MacLennan G, et al. Medical expulsive therapy in adults with ureteric colic: a multicentre, randomised, placebo-controlled trial. *Lancet.* 2015;386(9991):341.
17. Ye Z, Yang H, Li H, et al. A multicentre, prospective, randomized trial: comparative efficacy of tamsulosin and nifedipine in medical expulsive therapy for distal ureteric stones with renal colic. *BJU Int.* July 2011;108(2):276-279.
18. Worster AS, Bhanich Supapol W. Fluids and diuretics for acute ureteric colic. *Cochrane Database Syst Rev.* 15 February 2012;(2):CD004926.
19. Doluoglu ÖG, Demirbas A, Kilinc MF, et al. Can sexual intercourse be an alternative therapy for distal ureteral stones? A prospective, randomized, controlled study. *Urology.* July 2015;86(1):19-24.

51. LACERATION MANAGEMENT

1. Forsch RT. Essentials of skin laceration repair. *Am Fam Physician.* 15 October 2008;78(8):945-951.
2. Zehtabchi S, Tan A, Yadav K, Badawy A, Lucchesi M. The impact of wound age on the infection rate of simple lacerations repaired in the emergency department. *Injury.* November 2012;43(11):1793-1798.
3. Hollander JE, Singer AJ. Laceration management. *Ann Emerg Med.* 1999;34(3):356.
4. Perelman VS, Francis GJ, Rutledge T, et al. Sterile versus nonsterile gloves for repair of uncomplicated lacerations in the emergency department: a randomized controlled trial. *Ann Emerg Med.* March 2004; 43(3):362-370.
5. Fernandez R, Griffiths R. Water for wound cleansing. *Cochrane Database Syst Rev.* 23 January 2008;(1):CD003861.
6. Bruns TB, Worthington JM. Using tissue adhesive for wound repair. *Am Fam Physician.* 2000;61(5):1383-1388.
7. Quinn J, Wells G, Sutcliffe T, et al. A randomized trial comparing octylcyanoacrylate tissue adhesive and sutures in the management of lacerations. *JAMA.* 1997;277(19):1527-1530.
8. Quinn J, Cummings S, Callaham M, Sellers K. Suturing versus conservative management of lacerations of the hand: randomised controlled trial. *BMJ.* 10 August 2002;325(7359):299.
9. Ud-din Z, Aslam M, Gull S. Towards evidence based emergency medicine: best BETs from the Manchester Royal Infirmary. Should minor mucosal tongue lacerations be sutured in children? *Emerg Med J.* February 2007;24(2):123-124.
10. Lamell CW, Fraone G, Casamassimo PS, Wilson, S. Presenting characteristics and treatment outcomes for tongue lacerations in children. *Pediatr Dent.* 1999;21(1):34.

11. Cummings P, Del Beccaro MA. Antibiotics to prevent infection of simple wounds: a meta-analysis of randomized studies. *Am J Emerg Med.* 1995;13:396-400.

52. MEASLES (RUBEOLA)

1. Richardson M, Elliman D, Maguire H, Simpson J, Nicoll A. Evidence base of incubation periods, periods of infectiousness and exclusion policies for the control of communicable diseases in schools and preschools. *Pediatr Infect Dis J.* 2001;20(4):380.
2. Moss WJ, Griffin DE. Measles. *Lancet.* 14 January 2012;379(9811):153-164.
3. Rosen JB, Rota JS, Hickman CJ, et al. Outbreak of measles among persons with prior evidence of immunity, New York City, 2011. *Clin Infect Dis.* May 2014;58(9):1205-1210.
4. Steichen O, Dautheville S. Koplik spots in early measles. *CMAJ.* 3 March 2009; 180(5):583.
5. Abramson O, Dagan R, Tal A, Sofer S. Severe complications of measles requiring intensive care in infants and young children. *Arch Pediatr Adolesc Med.* 1995;149(11):1237.
6. Cherry JD. Measles virus. In: Feigin RD, Cherry JD, Demmler-Harrison GJ, et al., eds. *Textbook of Pediatric Infectious Diseases.* 6th ed. Philadelphia, PA: Saunders, 2009:2427.
7. Goodson JL, Seward JF. Measles 50 years after use of measles vaccine. *Infect Dis Clin North Am.* December 2015;29(4):725-743.
8. De Swart RL, Nur Y, Abdallah A, et al. Combination of reverse transcriptase PCR analysis and immunoglobulin M detection on filter paper blood samples allows diagnostic and epidemiological studies of measles. *J Clin Microbiol.* January 2001;39(1):270-273.
9. Ramsay M, Reacher M, O'Flynn C, et al. Causes of morbilliform rash in a highly immunised English population. *Arch Dis Child.* September 2002;87(3):202-206.
10. Atkinson W, Wolfe C, Hamborsky J, eds. *Epidemiology and Prevention of Vaccine-Preventable Diseases* (The Pink Book).12th ed. Washington, DC: The Public Health Foundation, 2011.
11. Atmar RL, Englund JA, Hammill H. Complications of measles during pregnancy. *Clin Infect Dis.* 1992;14(1):217.
12. Huiming Y, Chaomin W, Meng M. Vitamin A for treating measles in children. *Cochrane Database Syst Rev.* 19 October 2005;(4):CD001479.

53. ORBITAL CELLULITIS

1. Hauser A, Fogarasi S. Periorbital and orbital cellulitis. *Pediatr Rev.* June 2010;31(6):242-249.
2. Chandler JR, Langenbrunner DJ, Stevens ER. The pathogenesis of orbital complications in acute sinusitis. *Laryngoscope.* September 1970;80(9):1414-1428.
3. Zhang J, Stringer MD. Ophthalmic and facial veins are not valveless. *Clin Exp Ophthalmol.* 2010;38(5):502.
4. Nageswaran S, Woods CR, Benjamin DK Jr, Givner LB, Shetty AK. Orbital cellulitis in children. *Pediatr Infect Dis J.* 2006;25(8):695.

5. Uzcátegui N, Warman R, Smith A, Howard CW. Clinical practice guidelines for the management of orbital cellulitis. *J Pediatr Ophthalmol Strabismus.* 1998;35(2):73.
6. Sobol SE, Marchand J, Tewfik TL, Manoukian JJ, Schloss MD. Orbital complications of sinusitis in children. *J Otolaryngol.* 2002;31(3):131.
7. Mahalingam-Dhingra A, Lander L, Preciado DA, Taylormoore J, Shah RK. Orbital and periorbital infections: a national perspective. *Arch Otolaryngol Head Neck Surg.* 2011;137(8):769.
8. Pushker N, Tejwani LK, Bajaj MS, Khurana S, Velpandian T, Chandra M. Role of oral corticosteroids in orbital cellulitis. *Am J Ophthalmol.* July 2013;156(1):178-183.

54. ORGANOPHOSPHATE

1. Holstege CP, Borek HA. Toxidromes. *Crit Care Clin.* October 2012;28(4):479-498.
2. Indira M, Andrews MA, Rakesh TP. Incidence, predictors, and outcome of intermediate syndrome in cholinergic insecticide poisoning: a prospective observational cohort study.*Clin Toxicol* (Phila). 2013;51(9):838.
3. Johnson, MK. Mechanisms of and biomarkers for acute and delayed neuropathic effects of organophosphorus esters. In: Amaral-Mendes, J, Traviseds, CC eds. *Use of Biomarkers in Assessing Health and Environmental Impact of Chemical Pollutants. NATO Advanced Study Workshop.* Luso, Portugal: Plenum Press, 1993:169.
4. Levine M, Brooks DE, Truitt CA, Wolk BJ, Boyer EW, Ruha AM. Toxicology in the ICU: Part 1: general overview and approach to treatment. *Chest.* September 2011;140(3):795-806.
5. Eddleston M, Roberts D, Buckley N. Management of severe organophosphorus pesticide poisoning. *Crit Care.* 2002;6(3):259.
6. Johnson MK, Jacobsen D, Meredith TJ, et al. Evaluation of antidotes for poisoning by organophosphorus pesticides. *Emerg Med.* 2000;12:22.
7. Eyer P. The role of oximes in the management of organophosphorus pesticide poisoning. *Toxicol Rev.* 2003;22(3):165.
8. Schier JG, Hoffman RS. Treatment of sarin exposure. *JAMA.* 2004;291(2):182.
9. Eddleston M, Szinicz L, Eyer P, Buckley N. Oximes in acute organophosphorus pesticide poisoning: a systematic review of clinical trials. *QJM.* 2002;95(5):275.
10. Pawar KS, Bhoite RR, Pillay CP, Chavan SC, Malshikare DS, Garad SG. Continuous pralidoxime infusion versus repeated bolus injection to treat organophosphorus pesticide poisoning: a randomised controlled trial. *Lancet.* 2006;368(9553):2136.
11. Tuovinen K. Organophosphate-induced convulsions and prevention of neuropathological damages. *Toxicology.* 2004;196(1-2):31.
12. Tunnicliff G. Basis of the antiseizure action of phenytoin. *Gen Pharmacol.* 1996; 27:1091-1097.
13. Chen HY, Albertson TE, Olson KR. Treatment of drug-induced seizures. *Br J Clin Pharmacol.* September 2015;81(3):412-419.
14. Eddleston M, Juszczak E, Buckley NA, et al. Multiple-dose activated charcoal in acute self-poisoning: a randomised controlled trial. *Lancet.* 2008;371(9612):579.

55. PANCREATITIS

1. Tenner S, Baillie J, DeWitt J, Vege SS. American College of Gastroenterology guideline: management of acute pancreatitis. *Am J Gastroenterol.* September 2013;108(9):1400-1415; 1416.
2. Braganza JM, Lee SH, McCloy RF, McMahon MJ. Chronic pancreatitis. *Lancet.* 2 April 2011;377(9772):1184-1197.
3. Swaroop VS, Chari ST, Clain JE. Severe acute pancreatitis. *JAMA.* 2004;291(23):2865.
4. Banks PA, Freeman ML. Practice guidelines in acute pancreatitis. *Am J Gastroenterol.* 2006;101(10):2379.
5. Mookadam F, Cikes M. Images in clinical medicine. Cullen's and Turner's signs. *N Engl J Med.* September 2005;353(13):1386.
6. Marinella MA. Cullen's sign associated with metastatic thyroid cancer. *N Engl J Med.* 14 January 1999;340(2):149-150.
7. Banks PA, Bollen TL, Dervenis C, et al. Classification of acute pancreatitis—2012: revision of the Atlanta classification and definitions by international consensus. *Gut.* January 2013;62(1):102-111.
8. Yadav D, Agarwal N, Pitchumoni CS. A critical evaluation of laboratory tests in acute pancreatitis. *Am J Gastroenterol.* 2002;97(6):1309.
9. Rompianesi G, Hann A, Komolafe O, Pereira SP, Davidson BR, Gurusamy KS. Serum amylase and lipase and urinary trypsinogen and amylase for diagnosis of acute pancreatitis. *Cochrane Database Syst Rev.* 21 April 2017;4:CD012010.
10. Gumaste VV, Dave PB, Weissman D, Messer J. Lipase/amylase ratio. A new index that distinguishes acute episodes of alcoholic from nonalcoholic acute pancreatitis. *Gastroenterology.* November 1991;101(5):1361-1366.
11. Tenner S, Dubner H, Steinberg W. Predicting gallstone pancreatitis with laboratory parameters: a meta-analysis. *Am J Gastroenterol.* October 1994;89(10):1863-1866.
12. Ranson JH, Turner JW, Roses DF, Rifkind KM, Spencer FC. Respiratory complications in acute pancreatitis. *Ann Surg.* 1974;179(5):557.
13. Johnson C, Charnley R, Rowlands B, et al. UK guidelines for the management of acute pancreatitis. *Gut.* 2005;54 (3 Suppl):1.
14. Haydock MD, Mittal A, Wilms HR, Phillips A, Petrov MS, Windsor JA. Fluid therapy in acute pancreatitis: anybody's guess. *Ann Surg.* 2013;257(2):182.
15. Wu BU, Hwang JQ, Gardner TH, et al. Lactated ringer's solution reduces systemic inflammation compared with saline in patients with acute pancreatitis. *Clin Gastroenterol Hepatol.* 2011;9(8):710.
16. Ona XB, Comas DR, Urrútia G. Opioids for acute pancreatitis pain. *Cochrane Database Syst Rev.* 26 July 2013;(7):CD009179.
17. Helm JF, Venu RP, Geenen JE, et al. Effects of morphine on the human sphincter of Oddi. *Gut.* 1988;29(10):1402.
18. Tenner S, Baillie J, DeWitt J, Vege SS. American College of Gastroenterology guideline: management of acute pancreatitis. *Am J Gastroenterol.* 2013;108(9):1400.

19. AGA Institute Governing Board. AGA Institute medical position statement on acute pancreatitis. *Gastroenterology.* May 2007;132(5):2019-2021.
20. Working Group IAP/APA Acute Pancreatitis Guidelines. IAP/APA evidence-based guidelines for the management of acute pancreatitis. *Pancreatology.* July-August 2013;13 (4 Suppl 2):e1-e15.
21. Wu BU, Banks PA. Clinical management of patients with acute pancreatitis. *Gastroenterology.* June 2013;144(6):1272-1281.

56. PERITONSILLAR ABSCESS

1. Schraff S, McGinn JD, Derkay CS. Peritonsillar abscess in children: a 10-year review of diagnosis and management. *Int J Pediatr Otorhinolaryngol.* 2001;57(3):213.
2. Baldassari C, Shah RK. Pediatric peritonsillar abscess: an overview. *Infect Disord Drug Targets.* 12 August 2012;12(4):277-280.
3. Szuhay G, Tewfik TL. Peritonsillar abscess or cellulitis? A clinical comparative paediatric study. *J Otolaryngol.* 1998;27(4):206.
4. Powell J, Wilson JA. An evidence-based review of peritonsillar abscess. *Clin Otolaryngol.* April 2012;37(2):136-145.
5. Bandarkar AN, Adeyiga AO, Fordham MT, Preciado D, Reilly BK. Tonsil ultrasound: technical approach and spectrum of pediatric peritonsillar infections. *Pediatr Radiol.* June 2016;46(7):1059-1067.
6. Repanos C, Mukherjee P, Alwahab Y. Role of microbiological studies in management of peritonsillar abscess. *J Laryngol Otol.* August 2009;123(8):877-879.
7. Simons JP, Branstetter BF IV, Mandell DL. Bilateral peritonsillar abscesses: case report and literature review. *Am J Otolaryngol.* 2006;27(6):443.
8. Beahm ED, Elden LM. Bacterial infections of the neck. In: Burg FD, Ingelfinger JR, Polin RA, et al., eds. *Current Pediatric Therapy.* 18th ed. Philadelphia, PA: Saunders, 2006:1117.
9. Ban MJ, Nam Y, Park JH. Detection of peritonsillar abscess using smartphone-based thermal imaging. *Pak J Med Sci.* March-April 2017; 33(2):502-504.
10. Goldstein NA, Hammerschlag MR. Peritonsillar, retropharyngeal, and parapharyngeal abscesses. In: Feigin RD, Cherry JD, Demmler-Harrison GJ, et al, eds. *Textbook of Pediatric Infection Diseases.* 6th ed. Philadelphia, PA: Saunders, 2009:177.
11. Galioto NJ. Peritonsillar abscess. *Am Fam Physician.* 15 April 2017;95(8):501-506.
12. Johnson RF, Stewart MG, Wright CC. An evidence-based review of the treatment of peritonsillar abscess. *Otolaryngol Head Neck Surg.* 2003;128(3):332.
13. Yellon RF. Head and neck space infections. In: Bluestone CD, Casselbrant ML, Stool SE, et al., eds. *Pediatric Otolaryngology.* 4th ed. Philadelphia, PA: Saunders, 2003:1681.
14. Brodsky L, Sobie SR, Korwin D, Stanievich JF. A clinical prospective study of peritonsillar abscess in children. *Laryngoscope.* 1988;98(7):780.
15. Kim DK, Lee JW, Na YS, Kim MJ, Lee JH, Park CH. Clinical factor for successful nonsurgical treatment of pediatric peritonsillar abscess. *Laryngoscope.* 2015;125(11):2608.

16. Apostolopoulos NJ, Nikolopoulos TP, Bairamis TN. Peritonsillar abscess in children. Is incision and drainage an effective management? *Int J Pediatr Otorhinolaryngol.* 1995;31(2-3):129.
17. Ozbek C, Aygenc E, Tuna EU, Selcuk A, Ozdem C. Use of steroids in the treatment of peritonsillar abscess. *J Laryngol Otol.* 2004;118(6):439.
18. Hur K, Zhou S, Kysh L. Adjunct steroids in the treatment of peritonsillar abscess: a systematic review. *Laryngoscope.* May 2017;31:1-6.
19. Lamkin RH, Portt J. An outpatient medical treatment protocol for peritonsillar abscess. *Ear Nose Throat J.* October 2006;85(10):658; 660.

57. PNEUMONIA (COMMUNITY ACQUIRED)

1. Metlay JP, Fine MJ. Testing strategies in the initial management of patients with community-acquired pneumonia. *Ann Intern Med.* 2003;138(2):109.
2. Metlay JP, Kapoor WN, Fine MJ. Does this patient have community-acquired pneumonia? Diagnosing pneumonia by history and physical examination. *JAMA.* 1997;278(17):1440.
3. Watkins RR, Lemonovich TL. Diagnosis and management of community-acquired pneumonia in adults. *Am Fam Physician.* 1 June 2011;83(11):1299-1306.
4. Mandell LA, Wunderink RG, Anzueto A, et al. Infectious Diseases Society of America/American Thoracic Society consensus guidelines on the management of community-acquired pneumonia in adults. *Clin Infect Dis.* 1 March 2007;44 (2 Suppl) :S27-72.
5. Self WH, Balk RA, Grijalva CG, et al. Procalcitonin as a marker of etiology in adults hospitalized with community-acquired pneumonia. *Clin Infect Dis.* 15 July 2017;65(2):183-190.
6. Bafadhel M, Clark TW, Reid C, et al. Procalcitonin and C-reactive protein in hospitalized adult patients with community-acquired pneumonia or exacerbation of asthma or COPD. *Chest.* June 2011;139(6):1410-1418.
7. Schuetz P, Müller B, Christ-Crain M, et al. Procalcitonin to initiate or discontinue antibiotics in acute respiratory tract infections. *Cochrane Database Syst Rev.* 12 September 2012;(9):CD007498.
8. Campbell SG, Marrie TJ, Anstey R, Dickinson G, Ackroyd-Stolarz S. The contribution of blood cultures to the clinical management of adult patients admitted to the hospital with community-acquired pneumonia: a prospective observational study. *Chest.* 2003;123(4):1142.
9. The British Thoracic Society. Guidelines for the management of community-acquired pneumonia in adults admitted to hospital. *Br J Hosp Med.* 3-16 March 1993;49(5):346-350.

58. PREECLAMPSIA

1. American College of Obstetricians and Gynecologists. Hypertension in pregnancy. *Obstet Gynecol.* November 2013;122(5):1122-1131.

2. Cunningham FG, Lindheimer MD. Hypertension in pregnancy. *N Engl J Med.* 1992;326(14):927.
3. Leeman L, Fontaine P. Hypertensive disorders of pregnancy. *Am Fam Physician.* 1 July 2008;78(1):93-100.
4. Odegård RA, Vatten LJ, Nilsen ST, Salvesen KA, Austgulen R. Preeclampsia and fetal growth. *Obstet Gynecol.* 2000;96(6):950.
5. Thangaratinam S, Ismail KM, Sharp S, Coomarasamy A, Khan KS; Tests in Prediction of Pre-eclampsia Severity review group. Accuracy of serum uric acid in predicting complications of pre-eclampsia: a systematic review. *BJOG.* April 2006;113(4): 369-378.
6. Magee LA, Pels A, Helewa M, et al. Diagnosis, evaluation, and management of the hypertensive disorders of pregnancy: executive summary. *J Obstet Gynaecol Can.* May 2014;36(5):416-441.
7. Hauth JC, Ewell MG, Levine RJ, et al. Pregnancy outcomes in healthy nulliparas who developed hypertension. Calcium for Preeclampsia Prevention Study Group. *Obstet Gynecol.* 2000;95(1):24.
8. Waugh J, Bosio P, Shennan A, Halligan A. Inpatient monitoring on an outpatient basis: managing hypertensive pregnancies in the community using automated technologies. *J Soc Gynecol Investig.* January 2001;8(1):14-17.
9. Barton JR, Istwan NB, Rhea D, Collins A, Stanziano GJ. Cost-savings analysis of an outpatient management program for women with pregnancy-related hypertensive conditions. *Dis Manag.* 2006;9(4):236.
10. Turnbull DA, Wilkinson C, Gerard K, et al. Clinical, psychosocial, and economic effects of antenatal day care for three medical complications of pregnancy: a randomised controlled trial of 395 women. *Lancet.* 2004;363(9415):1104.
11. Berhan Y, Berhan A. Should magnesium sulfate be administered to women with mild pre-eclampsia? A systematic review of published reports on eclampsia. *J Obstet Gynaecol Res.* 2015;41(6):831.
12. Sibai BM. Magnesium sulfate prophylaxis in preeclampsia: lessons learned from recent trials. *Am J Obstet Gynecol.* 2004;190(6):1520.
13. Al-Safi Z, Imudia AN, Filetti LC, Hobson DT, Bahado-Singh RO, Awonuga AO. Delayed postpartum preeclampsia and eclampsia: demographics, clinical course, and complications. *Obstet Gynecol.* November 2011;118(5):1102-1107.
14. Sibai BM. Diagnosis, prevention, and management of eclampsia. *Obstet Gynecol.* 2005;105(2):402.
15. Lindenstrøm E, Boysen G, Nyboe J. Influence of systolic and diastolic blood pressure on stroke risk: a prospective observational study. *Am J Epidemiol.* 1995;142(12):1279.
16. Sibai BM. Magnesium sulfate prophylaxis in preeclampsia: lessons learned from recent trials. *Am J Obstet Gynecol.* 2004;190(6):1520.
17. Delgado-Escueta AV, Wasterlain C, Treiman DM, Porter RJ. Current concepts in neurology: management of status epilepticus. *N Engl J Med.* 1982;306(22):1337.

59. PROCEDURAL CONSCIOUS SEDATION

1. American Society of Anesthesiologists Task Force on Sedation and Analgesia by Non-Anesthesiologists. Practice guidelines for sedation and analgesia by non-anesthesiologists. *Anesthesiology.* 2002;96(4):1004.
2. Miller MA, Levy P, Patel MM. Procedural sedation and analgesia in the emergency department: what are the risks? *Emerg Med Clin North Am.* 2005;23(2):551.
3. Gan TJ. Pharmacokinetic and pharmacodynamic characteristics of medications used for moderate sedation. *Clin Pharmacokinet.* 2006;45(9):855.
4. Godwin SA, Burton JH, Gerardo CJ, et al. Clinical policy: procedural sedation and analgesia in the emergency department. *Ann Emerg Med.* February 2014;63(2):247-258.
5. Miner JR, Burton JH. Clinical practice advisory: emergency department procedural sedation with propofol. *Ann Emerg Med.* 2007;50(2):182.
6. Lamperti M. Adult procedural sedation: an update. *Curr Opin Anaesthesiol.* December 2015;28(6):662-667.
7. Swanson ER, Seaberg DC, Mathias S. The use of propofol for sedation in the emergency department. *Acad Emerg Med.* 1996;3(3):234.
8. Miner JR, Danahy M, Moch A, Biros M. Randomized clinical trial of etomidate versus propofol for procedural sedation in the emergency department. *Ann Emerg Med.* 2007;49(1):15.
9. Horn E, Nesbit SA. Pharmacology and pharmacokinetics of sedatives and analgesics. *Gastrointest Endosc Clin N Am.* 2004;14(2):247.
10. Bahn EL, Holt KR. Procedural sedation and analgesia: a review and new concepts. *Emerg Med Clin North Am.* 2005;23(2):503.
11. Newman DH, Azer MM, Pitetti RD, Singh S. When is a patient safe for discharge after procedural sedation? The timing of adverse effect events in 1367 pediatric procedural sedations. *Ann Emerg Med.* 2003;42(5):627.

60. PULMONARY EMBOLISM

1. Goldhaber SZ, Grodstein F, Stampfer MJ, et al. A prospective study of risk factors for pulmonary embolism in women. *JAMA.* 1997;277(8):642.
2. Busse LW, Vourlekis JS. Submassive pulmonary embolism. *Crit Care Clin.* July 2014;30(3):447-473.
3. Konstantinides SV, Torbicki A, Agnelli G, et al. 2014 ESC guidelines on the diagnosis and management of acute pulmonary embolism. *Eur Heart J.* 14 November 2014;35(43):3033-3069, 3069a-3069k.
4. van Belle A, Büller HR, Huisman MV, et al. Effectiveness of managing suspected pulmonary embolism using an algorithm combining clinical probability, D-dimer testing, and computed tomography. *JAMA.* 2006;295:172.
5. Stein PD, Beemath A, Matta F, et al. Clinical characteristics of patients with acute pulmonary embolism: data from PIOPED II. *Am J Med.* October 2007;120(10):871-879.

6. Raja AS, Greenberg JO, Qaseem A, et al. Evaluation of patients with suspected acute pulmonary embolism: best practice advice from the Clinical Guidelines Committee of the American College of Physicians. *Ann Intern Med.* 2015;163(9):701.
7. Chan WS, Ray JG, Murray S, Coady GE, Coates G, Ginsberg JS. Suspected pulmonary embolism in pregnancy: clinical presentation, results of lung scanning, and subsequent maternal and pediatric outcomes. *Arch Intern Med.* 2002;162(10):1170.
8. Leung AN, Bull TM, Jaeschke R, et al. An official American Thoracic Society/Society of Thoracic Radiology clinical practice guideline: evaluation of suspected pulmonary embolism in pregnancy. *Am J Respir Crit Care Med.* 2011; 184:1200.
9. Guyatt GH, Akl EA, Crowther M, Gutterman DD, Schuünemann HJ; American College of Chest Physicians Antithrombotic Therapy and Prevention of Thrombosis Panel. Executive summary: antithrombotic therapy and prevention of thrombosis, 9th ed: American College of Chest Physicians evidence-based clinical practice guidelines. *Chest.* February 2012;141(2 Suppl):7S-47S.

61. PYELONEPHRITIS

1. Hooton TM. Clinical practice. Uncomplicated urinary tract infection. *N Engl J Med.* 15 March 2012;366(11):1028-1037.
2. Gupta K, Hooton TM, Naber KG, et al. International clinical practice guidelines for the treatment of acute uncomplicated cystitis and pyelonephritis in women: a 2010 update by the Infectious Diseases Society of America and the European Society for Microbiology and Infectious Diseases. *Clin Infect Dis.* 1 March 2011;52(5):e103-120.
3. Fairley KF, Carson NE, Gutch RC, et al. Site of infection in acute urinary-tract infection in general practice. *Lancet.* 1971;2(7725):615.
4. Colgan R, Williams M. Diagnosis and treatment of acute uncomplicated cystitis. *Am Fam Physician.* 1 October 2011;84(7):771-776.
5. Johnson JR, Vincent LM, Wang K, Roberts PL, Stamm WE. Renal ultrasonographic correlates of acute pyelonephritis. *Clin Infect Dis.* 1992;14(1):15.
6. Kawashima A, LeRoy AJ. Radiologic evaluation of patients with renal infections. *Infect Dis Clin North Am.* 2003;17(2):433.
7. Fihn SD. Clinical practice. Acute uncomplicated urinary tract infection in women. *N Engl J Med.* 17 July 2003;349(3):259-266.
8. MacFadden DR, Ridgway JP, Robicsek A, Elligsen M, Daneman N. Predictive utility of prior positive urine cultures. *Clin Infect Dis.* November 2014;59(9):1265-1271.
9. Peterson J, Kaul S, Khashab M, Fisher AC, Kahn JB. A double-blind, randomized comparison of levofloxacin 750 mg once-daily for five days with ciprofloxacin 400/500 mg twice-daily for 10 days for the treatment of complicated urinary tract infections and acute pyelonephritis. *Urology.* 2008;71(1):17.
10. Jepson RG, Mihaljevic L, Craig J. Cranberries for treating urinary tract infections. *Cochrane Database Syst Rev.* 2000;(2):CD001322.

11. Ramakrishnan K, Scheid DC. Diagnosis and management of acute pyelonephritis in adults. *Am Fam Physician.* 1 March 2005;71(5):933-942.
12. Foxman B, Klemstine KL, Brown PD. Acute pyelonephritis in US hospitals in 1997: hospitalization and in-hospital mortality. *Ann Epidemiol.* February 2003;13(2):144-150.

62. RABIES: MAMMAL BITES

1. Oehler, RL, Velez AP, Mizrachi M, Lamarche J, Gompf S. Bite-related and septic syndromes caused by cats and dogs. *Lancet Infect Dis.* July 2009;9(7):439-447.
2. Talan DA, Ciltron DM, Abrahamian F, Moran GJ, Goldstein EJ. Bacteriologic analysis of infected dog and cat bites. Emergency Medicine Animal Bite Infection Study Group. *N Engl J Med.* 14 January 1999;340(2):85-92.
3. Talan DA, Ciltron DM, Abrahamian F, et al. Clinical presentation and bacteriologic analysis of infected human bites in patients presenting to emergency departments. *Clin Infect Dis.* 1 December 2003;37(11):1481-1489.
4. Brook, J. 2009. Management of human and animal bite wound infection: an overview. *Curr Infect Dis Rep.* September 2009;11(5):389-395.
5. Iannelli A, Lupi G. Penetrating brain injuries from a dog bite in an infant. *Pediatr Neurosurg.* 2005;41(1):41.
6. Fleisher, kGR. The management of bite wounds. *N Engl J Med.* 14 January 1999;340(2):138-140.
7. Stevens DL, Bisno AL, Chambers HF, et al. Infectious Diseases Society of America. Practice guidelines for the diagnosis and management of skin and soft-tissue infections. *Clin Infect Dis.* 15 November 2005;41(10):1373-1496.
8. Stevens DL, Bisno AL, Chambers HF, et al. Practice guidelines for the diagnosis and management of skin and soft tissue infections. *Clin Infect Dis.* 15 November 2005;41(10):1373-1406.

63. RADIAL HEAD SUBLUXATION

1. Welch R, Chounthirath T, Smith GA. Radial head subluxation among young children in the United States associated with consumer products and recreational activities. *Clin Pediatr.* (Phila). 2017;56(8):707.
2. Macias CG, Wiebe R, Bothner J. History and radiographic findings associated with clinically suspected radial head subluxations. *Pediatr Emerg Care.* 2000;16(1):22.
3. Krul M, van der Wouden JC, van Suijlekom-Smit LW, et al. Manipulative interventions for reducing pulled elbow in young children. *Cochrane Database Syst Rev.* 18 January 2012;1:CD007759.
4. Macias CG, Bothner J, Wiebe R. A comparison of supination/flexion to hyperpronation in the reduction of radial head subluxations. *Pediatrics.* 1998;102(1):e10.

64. RAPID SEQUENCE INTUBATION (RSI)

1. Ramachandran SK, Cosnowski A, Shanks A, Turner CR. Apneic oxygenation during prolonged laryngoscopy in obese patients: a randomized, controlled trial of nasal oxygen administration. *J Clin Anesth.* 2010;22(3):164.
2. Sagarin MJ, Barton ED, Chng YM, Walls RM; National Emergency Airway Registry Investigators. Airway management by US and Canadian emergency medicine residents: a multicenter analysis of more than 6,000 endotracheal intubation attempts. *Ann Emerg Med.* October 2005;46(4):328-336.
3. Pandit JJ, Duncan T, Robbins PA. Total oxygen uptake with two maximal breathing techniques and the tidal volume breathing technique: a physiologic study of preoxygenation. *Anesthesiology.* 2003;99(4):841.
4. Ding ZN, Shibata K, Yamamoto K, Kobayashi T, Murakami S. Decreased circulation time in the upper limb reduces the lag time of the finger pulse oximeter response. *Can J Anaesth.* January 1992;39(1):87-89.
5. Ellis DY, Harris T, Zideman D. Cricoid pressure in emergency department rapid sequence tracheal intubations: a risk-benefit analysis. *Ann Emerg Med.* 2007;50(6):653.

65. RESPIRATORY SYNCYTIAL VIRUS

1. American Academy of Pediatrics. Respiratory syncytial virus. In: Kimberlin DW, Brady MT, Jackson MA, et al, eds. *Red Book: 2015 Report of the Committee on Infectious Diseases.* 30th ed. Elk Grove Village, IL: American Academy of Pediatrics, 2015:667.
2. Hall CB, Weinberg GA, Iwane MK, et al. The burden of respiratory syncytial virus infection in young children. *N Engl J Med.* 2009;360(6):588.
3. Falsey AR, Walsh EE. Respiratory syncytial virus infection in adults. *Clin Microbiol Rev.* 2000;13(3):371.
4. Ralston SL, Lieberthal AS, Meissner HC, et al. Clinical practice guideline: the diagnosis, management, and prevention of bronchiolitis. *Pediatrics.* November 2014;134(5):e1474-e1502.
5. Hall CB, Walsh EE, Schnabel KC, et al. Occurrence of groups A and B of respiratory syncytial virus over 15 years: associated epidemiologic and clinical characteristics in hospitalized and ambulatory children. *J Infect Dis.* 1990;162(6):1283.
6. Erez DL, Yarden-Bilavsky H, Mendelson E, et al. Apnea induced by respiratory syncytial virus infection is not associated with viral invasion of the central nervous system. *Pediatr Infect Dis J.* 2014;33(8):880.
7. Uren EC, Williams AL, Jack I, Rees JW. Association of respiratory virus infections with sudden infant death syndrome. *Med J Aust.* 1980;1(9):417.
8. Purcell K, Fergie J. Lack of usefulness of an abnormal white blood cell count for predicting a concurrent serious bacterial infection in infants and young children hospitalized with respiratory syncytial virus lower respiratory tract infection. *Pediatr Infect Dis J.* April 2007;26(4):311-315.

9. Bordley WC, Viswanathan M, King VJ, et al. Diagnosis and testing in bronchiolitis: a systematic review. *Arch Pediatr Adolesc Med.* February 2004;158(2):119-126.
10. Ralston S, Hill V, Waters A. Occult serious bacterial infection in infants younger than 60 to 90 days with bronchiolitis: a systematic review. *Arch Pediatr Adolesc Med.* October 2011;165(10):951-956.
11. Hartling L, Bialy LM, Vandermeer B, et al. Epinephrine for bronchiolitis. *Cochrane Database Syst Rev.* 15 June 2011;(6):CD003123.
12. Blom D, Ermers M, Bont L, van Aalderen WM, van Woensel JB. Inhaled corticosteroids during acute bronchiolitis in the prevention of post-bronchiolitic wheezing. *Cochrane Database Syst Rev.* 24 January 2007;(1):CD004881.
13. Liu F, Ouyang J, Sharma AN, et al. Leukotriene inhibitors for bronchiolitis in infants and young children. *Cochrane Database Syst Rev.* 16 March 2015;(3):CD010636.
14. Sinha IP, McBride AK, Smith R, Fernandes RM. CPAP and high-flow nasal cannula oxygen in bronchiolitis. *Chest.* 2015;148(3):810.
15. Liet JM, Ducruet T, Gupta V, Cambonie G. Heliox inhalation therapy for bronchiolitis in infants. *Cochrane Database Syst Rev.* 18 September 2015;(9):CD006915.
16. Fernandes RM, Bialy LM, Vandermeer B, et al. Glucocorticoids for acute viral bronchiolitis in infants and young children. *Cochrane Database Syst Rev.* 4 June 2013;(6):CD004878.
17. Ricci V, Delgado Nunes V, Murphy MS, Cunningham S. Bronchiolitis in children: summary of NICE guidance. *BMJ.* 2 June 2015;350:h2305.
18. Bronchiolitis Guideline Team, Cincinnati Children's Hospital Medical Center. *Bronchiolitis pediatric evidence-based care guidelines* [2010; cited 24 February 2015]. www.cincinnatichildrens.org/service/j/anderson-center/evidence-based-care/recommendations/topic.
19. Mansbach JM, Clark S, Piedra PA, et al. Hospital course and discharge criteria for children hospitalized with bronchiolitis. *J Hosp Med.* April 2015;10(4):205-211.

66. ROCKY MOUNTAIN SPOTTED FEVER

1. Dahlgren FS, Holman RC, Paddock CD, Callinan LS, McQuiston JH. Fatal Rocky Mountain spotted fever in the US, 1999 – 2007. *Am J Trop Med Hyg.* 1 April 2012; 86(4):713-719.
2. U.S. Department of Health and Human Services. *Rocky Mountain Spotted Fever (RMSF)* [Internet]. Centers for Disease Control and Prevention; [updated 26 June 2017; cited 26 July 2017]. https://www.cdc.gov/rmsf/index.html.
3. Hattwick MA, Retailliau H, O'Brien RJ, Slutzker M, Fontaine RE, Hanson B. Fatal Rocky Mountain spotted fever. *JAMA.* 1978;240:1499-1503.
4. Usatine RP, Sandy N. Dermatologic emergencies. *Am Fam Physician.* 2010;82(7):773.
5. Buckingham SC, Marshall GS, Schutze GE, et al. Clinical and laboratory features, hospital course, and outcome of Rocky Mountain spotted fever in children. *J Pediatr. February.* 2007;150(2):180-184.

6. Walker DH. Rocky Mountain spotted fever: a disease in need of microbiological concern. *Clin Microbiol Rev.* July 1989;2(3):227-240.
7. Pickering L, Baker C, Kimberlin D, Long S, eds. *Red Book: 2009 Report of the Committee on Infectious Diseases.* 28th ed. Elk Grove Village, IL: American Academy of Pediatrics; 2009: 573-575.
8. Herbert WN, Seeds JW, Koontz WL, Cefalo RC. Rocky Mountain spotted fever in pregnancy: differential diagnosis and treatment. *South Med J.* September 1982;75(9):1063-1066.
9. Purvis JJ, Edwards MS. Doxycycline use for rickettsial disease in pediatric patients. *Pediatr Infect Dis J.* 2000;19:871-874.
10. Huntzinger A. Guidelines for the diagnosis and treatment of tick-borne rickettsial diseases. *Am Fam Physician.* 1 July 2007;76(1):137-139.

67. RX DRUG DIVERSION

1. Rehm J, Marmet S, Anderson P, et al. Defining substance use disorders: do we really need more than heavy use? *Alcohol and Alcohol.* 1 November 2013;48(6):633-640.
2. Von Korff M, Dublin S, Walker RL, et al. The impact of opioid risk reduction initiatives on high-dose opioid prescribing for patients on chronic opioid therapy. *J Pain.* January 2016;17(1):101-110.
3. Ives TJ, Chelminski PR, Hammett-Stabler CA, et al. Predictors of opioid misuse in patients with chronic pain: a prospective cohort study. *BMC Health Serv Res.* 2006;6:46.
4. Liebschutz JM, Saitz R, Weiss RD, et al. Clinical factors associated with prescription drug use disorder in urban primary care patients with chronic pain. *J Pain.* 2010;11(11):1047.
5. Fleming MF, Balousek SL, Klessig CL, Mundt MP, Brown DD. Substance use disorders in a primary care sample receiving daily opioid therapy. *J Pain.* July 2007;8(7):573-582.
6. Chou R, Fanciullo GJ, Fine PG, et al. Clinical guidelines for the use of chronic opioid therapy in chronic noncancer pain. *J Pain.* 2009;10(2):113.
7. Dowell D, Haegerich TM, Chou R. CDC Guideline for prescribing opioids for chronic pain—United States, 2016. *MMWR Recomm Rep.* 2016;65(1):1.
8. Hegmann KT, Weiss MS, Bowden K, et al. ACOEM practice guidelines: opioids for treatment of acute, subacute, chronic, and postoperative pain. *J Occup Environ Med.* December 2014;56(12):e143-e159.
9. Blondell RD, Azadfard M, Wisniewski AM. Pharmacologic therapy for acute pain. *Am Fam Physician.* 1 June 2013;87(11):766-772.
10. Paulozzi LJ, Kilbourne EM, Shah NG, et al. A history of being prescribed controlled substances and risk of drug overdose death. *Pain Med.* January 2012;13(1):87-95.
11. Berge KH, Dillon KR, Sikkink KM, Taylor TK, Lanier WL. Diversion of drugs within health care facilities, a multiple-victim crime: patterns of diversion, scope, consequences, detection, and prevention. *Mayo Clin Proc.* July 2012; 87(7): 674-682.

68. SALICYLATE TOXICITY

1. American College of Medical Toxicology. Guidance document: management priorities in salicylate toxicity. *J Med Toxicol.* March 2015;11(1):149-152.
2. O'Malley GF. Emergency department management of the salicylate-poisoned patient. *Emerg Med Clin North Am.* 2007;25(2):333.
3. Dargan PI, Wallace CI, Jones AL. An evidence based flowchart to guide the management of acute salicylate (aspirin) overdose. *Emerg Med J.* May 2002;19(3):206-209.
4. Hill JB. Salicylate intoxication. *N Engl J Med.* 1973;288(21):1110.
5. Greenberg MI, Hendrickson RG, Hofman M. Deleterious effects of endotracheal intubation in salicylate poisoning. *Ann Emerg Med.* 2003;41(4):583.
6. Leatherman JW, Schmitz PG. Fever, hyperdynamic shock, and multiple-system organ failure. A pseudo-sepsis syndrome associated with chronic salicylate intoxication. *Chest.* 1991;100(5):1391.
7. Barone JA, Raia JJ, Huang YC. Evaluation of the effects of multiple-dose activated charcoal on the absorption of orally administered salicylate in a simulated toxic ingestion model. *Ann Emerg Med.* 1988;17(1):34.
8. Proudfoot AT, Krenzelok EP, Vale JA. Position Paper on urine alkalinization. *J Toxicol Clin Toxicol.* 2004;42(1):1.
9. Thurston JH, Pollock PG, Warren SK, Jones EM. Reduced brain glucose with normal plasma glucose in salicylate poisoning. *J Clin Invest.* 1970;49(11):2139.
10. Juurlink DN, Gosselin S, Kielstein JT, et al. Extracorporeal treatment for salicylate poisoning: systematic review and recommendations from the EXTRIP workgroup. *Ann Emerg Med.* August 2015;66(2):165-181.

69. SEPSIS

1. Singer M, Deutschman CS, Seymour CW, et al. The third international consensus definitions for sepsis and septic shock (Sepsis-3). *JAMA.* 23 February 2016;315(8):801-810.
2. [No authors listed]. American College of Chest Physicians/Society of Critical Care Medicine Consensus Conference: definitions for sepsis and organ failure and guidelines for the use of innovative therapies in sepsis. *Crit Care Med.* 20 June 1992;20(6):864-874.
3. Sands KE, Bates DW, Lanken PN, et al. Epidemiology of sepsis syndrome in 8 academic medical centers. Academic Medical Center Consortium Sepsis Project Working Group *JAMA.* 1997;278(3):234.
4. Vincent JL, Bihari DJ, Suter PM, et al. The prevalence of nosocomial infection in intensive care units in Europe. Results of the European Prevalence of Infection in Intensive Care (EPIC) Study. EPIC International Advisory Committee. *JAMA.* 1995;274(8):639.
5. Jones GR, Lowes JA. The systemic inflammatory response syndrome as a predictor of bacteraemia and outcome from sepsis. *QJM.* 1996;89(7):515.
6. Seigel TA, Cocchi MN, Salciccioli J, et al. Inadequacy of temperature and white blood cell count in predicting bacteremia in patients with suspected infection. *J Emerg Med.* March 2012;42(3):254-259.

7. Dellinger RP, Levy MM, Rhodes A, et al. Surviving sepsis campaign: international guidelines for management of severe sepsis and septic shock: 2012. *Crit Care Me.* February 2013;41(2):580-637.
8. Vincent JL, Moreno R, Takala J, et al. The SOFA (Sepsis-related Organ Failure Assessment) score to describe organ dysfunction/failure. On behalf of the working group on sepsis-related problems of the European Society of Intensive Care Medicine. *Intensive Care Med.* July 1996;22(7):707-710.
9. Rhodes A, Evans LE, Alhazzani W, et al. Surviving Sepsis Campaign: international guidelines for management of sepsis and septic shock: 2016. *Intensive Care Med.* March 2017;43(3):304-377.
10. Fridkin SK, Hageman JC, Morrison M, et al. Methicillin-resistant staphylococcus aureus disease in three communities. Active Bacterial Core Surveillance Program of the Emerging Infections Program Network. *N Engl J Med.* 2005;352(14):1436.
11. Martin C, Papazian L, Perrin G, Saux P, Gouin F. Norepinephrine or dopamine for the treatment of hyperdynamic septic shock? *Chest.* 1993;103(6):1826.
12. Hollenberg SM, Ahrens TS, Annane D, et al. Practice parameters for hemodynamic support of sepsis in adult patients: 2004 update. *Crit Care Med.* 2004;32(9):1928.

70. SORE THROAT

1. Harris AM, Hicks LA, Qaseem A. Appropriate antibiotic use for acute respiratory tract infection in adults: advice for high-value care from the American College of Physicians and the Centers for Disease Control and Prevention. *Ann Intern Med.* 15 March 2016;164(6):425-434.
2. Centers for Disease Control and Prevention. *About diphtheria* [Internet]. National Center for Immunization and Respiratory Disease, Division of Bacterial Diseases; [updated 15 January 2016; cited 25 May 2017].https://www.cdc.gov/diphtheria/about/index.html.
3. Luzuriaga K, Sullivan JL. Infectious mononucleosis. *N Engl J Med* 2010;362(21):1993.
4. Huovinen P, Little P, Verheij T. Guideline for the management of acute sore throat. *Clin Microbiol Infect.* 2012;18 (1 Suppl):1.
5. Lathadevi HT, Karadi RN, Thobbi RV, Guggarigoudar SP, Kulkarni NH. Isolated uvulitis: an uncommon but not a rare clinical entity. *Indian J Otolaryngol Head Neck Surg.* April 2005;57(2):139-140.
6. Shulman ST, Bisno AL, Clegg HW, et al. Clinical practice guideline for the diagnosis and management of group A streptococcal pharyngitis: 2012 update by the Infectious Diseases Society of America. *Clin Infect Dis.* 15 November 2012;55(10):e86-e102.
7. Hayward GN, Hay AD, Moore MV, et al. Effect of oral dexamethasone without immediate antibiotics vs placebo on acute sore throat in adults. *JAMA.* 2017;317(15):1535-1543.
8. Korb K, Scherer M, Chenot JF. Steroids as adjuvant therapy for acute pharyngitis in ambulatory patients: a systematic review. *Ann Fam Med.* January 2010;8(1):58-63.
9. Tasar A, Yanturali S, Topacoglu H, Ersoy G, Unverir P, Sarikaya S. Clinical efficacy of dexamethasone for acute exudative pharyngitis. *J Emerg Med.* 2008;35(4):363-367.

10. Hayward G, Thompson MJ, Perera R, Glasziou PP, Del Mar CB, Heneghan CJ. Corticosteroids as standalone or add-on treatment for sore throat. *Cochrane Database Syst Rev.* 17 October 2012;10:CD008268.
11. Olsson B, Olsson B, Tibblin G. Effect of patients' expectations on recovery from acute tonsillitis. *Fam Pract.* September 1989;6(3):188-192.
12. Brook I, Gober AE. Persistence of group A beta-hemolytic streptococci in toothbrushes and removable orthodontic appliances following treatment of pharyngotonsillitis. *Arch Otolaryngol Head Neck Surg.* September 1998;124(9):993-995.
13. Kikuta H, Shibata M, Nakata S, et al. Efficacy of antibiotic prophylaxis for intrafamilial transmission of group A beta-hemolytic streptococci. *Pediatr Infect Dis J.* February 2007;26(2):139-141.
14. Gerber MA, Baltimore RS, Eaton CB, et al. Prevention of rheumatic fever and diagnosis and treatment of acute Streptococcal pharyngitis: a scientific statement from the American Heart Association Rheumatic Fever, Endocarditis, and Kawasaki Disease Committee of the Council on Cardiovascular Disease in the Young, the Interdisciplinary Council on Functional Genomics and Translational Biology, and the Interdisciplinary Council on Quality of Care and Outcomes Research: endorsed by the American Academy of Pediatrics. *Circulation.* 24 March 2009;119(11):1541-1551.

71. SUPERFICIAL THROMBOPHLEBITIS

1. Decousus H, Frappé P, Accassat S, et al. Epidemiology, diagnosis, treatment and management of superficial-vein thrombosis of the legs. *Best Pract Res Clin Haematol.* September 2012;25(3):275-284.
2. Cannegieter SC, Horváth-Puhó E, Schmidt M, et al. Risk of venous and arterial thrombotic events in patients diagnosed with superficial vein thrombosis: a nationwide cohort study. *Blood.* 2015;125(2):229.
3. Tait C, Baglin T, Watson H, et al. Guidelines on the investigation and management of venous thrombosis at unusual sites. *Br J Haematol.* October 2012;159(1):28-38.
4. Bernardi E, Camporese G, Büller HR, et al. Serial 2-point ultrasonography plus d-dimer vs whole-leg color-coded doppler ultrasonography for diagnosing suspected symptomatic deep vein thrombosis: a randomized controlled trial. *JAMA.* 2008;300(14):1653.
5. Blumenberg RM, Barton E, Gelfand ML, Skudder P, Brennan J. Occult deep venous thrombosis complicating superficial thrombophlebitis. *J Vasc Surg.* 1998;27(2):338.
6. Binder B, Lackner HK, Salmhofer W, Kroemer S, Custovic J, Hofmann-Wellenhof R.. Association between superficial vein thrombosis and deep vein thrombosis of the lower extremities. *Arch Dermatol.* 2009;145(7):753.
7. Guex JJ. Thrombotic complications of varicose veins. A literature review of the role of superficial venous thrombosis. *Dermatol Surg.* 1996;22(4):378.
8. Carrier M, Le Gal G, Wells PS, Fergusson D, Ramsay T, Rodger MA.. Systematic review: the Trousseau syndrome revisited: should we screen extensively for cancer in patients with venous thromboembolism? *Ann Intern Med.* 2008;149(5):323.

9. Cannegieter SC, Horváth-Puhó E, Schmidt M, et al. Risk of venous and arterial thrombotic events in patients diagnosed with superficial vein thrombosis: a nationwide cohort study. *Blood.* 8 January 2015;125(2):229-235.
10. Kearon C, Akl EA, Ornelas J, et al. Antithrombotic therapy for VTE disease: CHEST guideline and expert panel report. *Chest.* 2016;149(2):315.
11. Cosmi B. Management of superficial vein thrombosis. *J Thromb Haemost.* July 2015;13(7):1175-1183.
12. Decousus H, Prandoni P, Mismetti P, et al. Fondaparinux for the treatment of superficial-vein thrombosis in the legs. *N Engl J Med.* 23 September 2010;363(13):1222-1232.
13. Décousus H, Brégeault MF; Darmon JY, et al. A pilot randomized double-blind comparison of a low-molecular-weight heparin, a nonsteroidal anti-inflammatory agent, and placebo in the treatment of superficial vein thrombosis. *Arch Intern Med.* 28 July 2003;163(14):1657-1663.
14. Kalodiki E, Stvrtinova V, Allegra C, et al. Superficial vein thrombosis: a consensus statement. *Int Angiol.* June 2012;31(3):203-216.
15. Kearon C, Akl EA, Comerota AJ, et al. Antithrombotic therapy for VTE disease: Antithrombotic therapy and prevention of thrombosis, 9th ed: American College of Chest Physicians evidence-based clinical practice guidelines. *Chest.* February 2012;141(2 Suppl):e419S-e496S.

72. SYNCOPE

1. Soteriades ES, Evans JC, Larson MG, et al. Incidence and prognosis of syncope. *N Engl J Med.* 19 September 2002;347(12):878-885.
2. Jhanjee R, van Dijk JG, Sakaguchi S, Benditt DG. Syncope in adults: terminology, classification, and diagnostic strategy. *Pacing Clin Electrophysiol.* October 2006;29(10):1160-1169.
3. Linzer M, Yang EH, Estes NA 3rd, Wang P, Vorperian VR, Kapoor WN. Diagnosing syncope. Part 1: value of history, physical examination, and electrocardiography. Clinical Efficacy Assessment Project of the American College of Physicians. *Ann Intern Med.* 1997;126(12):989.
4. Shen WK, Sheldon RS, Benditt DG, et al. 2017 ACC/AHA/HRS guideline for the evaluation and management of patients with syncope: executive summary: a report of the American College of Cardiology/American Heart Association Task Force on clinical practice guidelines and the Heart Rhythm Society. *J Am Coll Cardiol.* 1 August 2017;70(5):620-663.
5. Gauer RL. Evaluation of syncope. *Am Fam Physician.* 15 September 2011;84(6):640-650.
6. American College of Physicians. *Five things physicians and patients should questions.* [Internet]. Choosing Wisely; [April 2012; cited 15 June 2017].http://www.choosingwisely.org/societies/american-college-of-physicians/.
7. Task Force for the Diagnosis and Management of Syncope; European Society of Cardiology (ESC); European Heart Rhythm Association (EHRA); Heart Failure Association (HFA); Heart Rhythm Society (HRS), Moya A, Sutton R, Ammirati F, et al.

Guidelines for the diagnosis and management of syncope (version 2009). *Eur Heart J.* November 2009;30(21):2631-2671.
8. Quinn JV, Stiell IG, McDermott DA, Sellers KL, Kohn MA, Wells GA. Derivation of the San Francisco Syncope Rule to predict patients with short-term serious outcomes. *Ann Emerg Med.* 2004;43(2):224.
9. Brignole M, Benditt DG. *Syncope: An Evidence-Based Approach.* New York, NY: Springer Science & Business Media, 2011:5.

73. TESTICULAR TORSION

1. Ta A, D'Arcy FT, Hoag N, D'Arcy JP, Lawrentschuk N. Testicular torsion and the acute scrotum: current emergency management. *Eur J Emerg Med.* June 2016;23(3):160-165.
2. Trojian TH, Lishnak TS, Heiman D. Epididymitis and orchitis: an overview. *Am Fam Physician.* 2009;79(7):583.
3. Molokwu CN, Somani BK, Goodman CM. Outcomes of scrotal exploration for acute scrotal pain suspicious of testicular torsion: a consecutive case series of 173 patients. *BJU Int.* 2011;107(6):990.
4. Livne PM, Sivan B, Karmazyn B, Ben-Meir D. Testicular torsion in the pediatric age group: diagnosis and treatment. *Pediatr Endocrinol Rev.* December 2003;1(2):128-133.
5. Rabinowitz R. The importance of the cremasteric reflex in acute scrotal swelling in children. *J Urol.* 1984;132(1):89.
6. Sharp VJ, Kieran K, Arlen AM. Testicular torsion: diagnosis, evaluation, and management. *Am Fam Physician.* 15 December 2013;88(12):835-840.
7. Pepe P, Panella P, Pennisi M, Aragona F. Does color oppler sonography improve the clinical assessment of patients with acute scrotum? *Eur J Radiol.* 2006;60(1):120.
8. Bowlin PR, Gatti JM, Murphy JP. Pediatric testicular torsion. *Surg Clin North Am.* February 2017;97(1):161-172.
9. Sheth KR, Keays M, Grimsby GM, et al. Diagnosing testicular torsion before urological consultation and imaging: validation of the TWIST score. *J Urol.* June 2016;195(6):1870-1876.
10. Sessions AE, Rabinowitz R, Hulbert WC, Goldstein MM, Mevorach RA. Testicular torsion: direction, degree, duration and disinformation. *J Urol.* 2003;169(2):663.
11. Kadish HA, Bolte RG. A retrospective review of pediatric patients with epididymitis, testicular torsion, and torsion of testicular appendages. *Pediatrics.* 1998;102(1 Pt 1):73.
12. Workowski KA, Bolan GA. Sexually transmitted diseases treatment guidelines, 2015. *MMWR Recomm Rep.* 5 June 2015;64(RR-03):1-137.

74. THREATENED ABORTION

1. Strobino B, Pantel-Silverman J. Gestational vaginal bleeding and pregnancy outcome. *Am J Epidemiol.* 1989;129(4):806.
2. Dighe M, Cuevas C, Moshiri M, Dubinsky T, Dogra VS. Sonography in first trimester bleeding. *J Clin Ultrasound.* 2008;36(6):352.

3. Von Stein GA, Munsick RA, Stiver K, Ryder K. Fetomaternal hemorrhage in threatened abortion. *Obstet Gynecol.* March 1992;79(3):383-386.
4. Deutchman M1, Tubay AT, Turok D. First trimester bleeding. *Am Fam Physician.* 1 June 2009;79(11):985-994.

75. THYROID STORM

1. Sarlis NJ, Gourgiotis L. Thyroid emergencies. *Rev Endocr Metab Disord.* 2003;4(2):129.
2. Burch HB, Wartofsky L. Life-threatening thyrotoxicosis. Thyroid storm. *Endocrinol Metab Clin North Am.* 1993;22(2):263.
3. Akamizu T, Satoh T, Isozaki O, et al. Diagnostic criteria, clinical features, and incidence of thyroid storm based on nationwide surveys. *Thyroid.* July 2012;22(7):661-679.
4. Chiha M, Samarasinghe S, Kabaker AS. Thyroid storm: an updated review. *J Intensive Care Med.* March 2015;30(3):131-140.

76. TOXIC INGESTION (ADULTS/PEDS)

1. Bryant S, Singer J. Management of toxic exposure in children. *Emerg Med Clin North Am.* 2003;21(1):101.
2. Mofenson HC, Greensher J. The unknown poison. *Pediatrics.* 1974;54(3):336.
3. McInerny TK, Adam HM, Campbell DE, et al., eds. *American Academy of Pediatrics Textbook of Pediatric Care.* 2nd ed. Elk Grove Village, IL: American Academy of Pediatrics, 2016.
4. Linden CH. General considerations in the evaluation and treatment of poisoning. In: Rippe JM, Irwin RS, Fink MP, et al, eds. *J Intensive Care Med.* Boston, MA: Little Brown and Company, 1996:1455.
5. Ratnapalan S, Potylitsina Y, Tan LH, Roifman M, Koren G. Measuring a toddler's mouthful: toxicologic considerations. *J Pediatr.* 2003;142(6):729.
6. Winter ML, Ellis MD, Snodgrass WR. Urine fluorescence using a Wood's lamp to detect the antifreeze additive sodium fluorescein: a qualitative adjunctive test in suspected ethylene glycol ingestions. *Ann Emerg Med.* 1990;19(6):663.
7. Woolf AD. Poisoning by unknown agents. *Pediatr Rev.* 1999;20(5):166.
8. Mofenson HC, Greensher J. The unknown poison. *Pediatrics.* 1974;54(3):336.
9. Pietrzak MP, Kuffner EK, Morgan DL, et al. Clinical policy for the initial approach to patients presenting with acute toxic ingestion or dermal or inhalation exposure. *Ann Emerg Med.* June 1999;33(6):735-761.
10. Hoffman RS, Goldfrank LR. The poisoned patient with altered consciousness. Controversies in the use of a 'coma cocktail'. *JAMA.* 1995;274(7):562.
11. Tran TP, Panacek EA, Rhee KJ, Foulke GE. Response to dopamine vs norepinephrine in tricyclic antidepressant-induced hypotension. *Acad Emerg Med.* 1997;4(9):864.
12. Hollander JE. The management of cocaine-associated myocardial ischemia. *N Engl J Med.* 1995;333(19):1267.

13. Battaglia J, Moss S, Rush J, et al. Haloperidol, lorazepam, or both for psychotic agitation? A multicenter, prospective, double-blind, emergency department study. *Am J Emerg Med.* 1997;15(4):335.
14. Blake KV, Massey KL, Hendeles L, Nickerson D, Neims A. Relative efficacy of phenytoin and phenobarbital for the prevention of theophylline-induced seizures in mice. *Ann Emerg Med.* 1988;17(10):1024.
15. Chyka PA, Seger D, Krenzelok EP, Vale JA; American Academy of Clinical Toxicology; European Association of Poisons Centres and Clinical Toxicologists. Position paper: single-dose activated charcoal. *Clin Toxicol* (Phila). 2005;43(2):61.
16. Vale JA, Kulig K, American Academy of Clinical Toxicology, European Association of Poisons Centres and Clinical Toxicologists. Position paper: gastric lavage. *J Toxicol Clin Toxicol.* 2004;42(7):933-943.
17. Dart RC, Borron SW, Caravati EM, et al. Expert consensus guidelines for stocking of antidotes in hospitals that provide emergency care. *Ann Emerg Med.* 2009;54(3):386.
18. Erickson TB, Thompson TM, Lu JJ. The approach to the patient with an unknown overdose. *Emerg Med Clin North Am.* May 2007;25(2):249-281; abstract vii.
19. Bryant S, Singer J. Management of toxic exposure in children. *Emerg Med Clin North Am.* 2003;21(1):101.
20. Brett AS, Rothschild N, Gray R, Perry M. Predicting the clinical course in intentional drug overdose. Implications for use of the intensive care unit. *Arch Intern Med.* 1987;147(1):133.
21. Lee HL, Lin HJ, Yeh ST, Chi CH, Guo HR. Presentations of patients of poisoning and predictors of poisoning-related fatality: findings from a hospital-based prospective study. *BMC Public Health.* 2008;8:7.

77. UPPER RESPIRATORY INFECTION

1. Kirkpatrick GL. The common cold. *Prim Care.* 1996;23(4):657.
2. Harris AM, Hicks LA, Qaseem A. Appropriate antibiotic use for acute respiratory tract infection in adults: advice for high-value care from the American College of Physicians and the Centers for Disease Control and Prevention. *Ann Intern Med.* 15 March 2016;164(6):425-434.
3. Altiner A, Wim S, Däubener W, et al. Sputum colour for diagnosis of a bacterial infection in patients with acute cough. *Scand J Prim Health Care.* 2009; 27(2):70-73.
4. Kaiser L, Lew D, Hirschel B, et al. Effects of antibiotic treatment in the subset of common-cold patients who have bacteria in nasopharyngeal secretions. *Lancet.* 1 June 1996;347(9014):1507-1510.
5. Simasek M, Blandino DA. Treatment of the common cold. *Am Fam Physician.* 15 February 2007;75(4):515-520.
6. Havas TE, Motbey JA, Gullane PJ. Prevalence of incidental abnormalities on computed tomographic scans of the paranasal sinuses. *Arch Otolaryngol Head Neck Surg.* 1988;114(8):856.

7. McBride TP, Doyle WJ, Hayden FG, Gwaltney JM Jr. Alterations of the eustachian tube, middle ear, and nose in rhinovirus infection. *Arch Otolaryngol Head Neck Surg.* 1989;115(9):1054.
8. Sharfstein JM, North M, Serwint JR. Over the counter but no longer under the radar—pediatric cough and cold medications. *N Engl J Med.* 2007;357(23):2321.
9. Singh M, Singh M, Jaiswal N, Chauhan A. Heated, humidified air for the common cold. *Cochrane Database Syst Rev.* 2017;8:CD001728.
10. Hayward G, Thompson MJ, Perera R, Del Mar CB, Glasziou PP, Heneghan CJ. Corticosteroids for the common cold. *Cochrane Database Syst Rev.* 13 October 2015;(10):CD008116.

78. URINARY RETENTION (AUR)

1. Selius BA, Subedi R. Urinary retention in adults: diagnosis & initial management. *Am Fam Physician.* 1 March 2008;77(5):643-650.
2. Choong S, Emberton M. Acute urinary retention. *BJU Int.* 2000:85(2):186-201.
3. Rosenstein D, McAninch JW. Urologic emergencies. *Med Clin North Am.* 2004;88(2):495-518.
4. D'Silva KA, Dahm P, Wong CL. Does this man with lower urinary tract symptoms have bladder outlet obstruction?: the Rational Clinical Examination: a systemic review. *JAMA.* 6 August 2014;312(5):535.
5. Stevens E. Bladder ultrasound: avoiding unnecessary catherizations. *Medsurg Nurs.* 2005;14(4):249-253.
6. Nyman MA, Schwenk NM, Silverstein MD. Management of urinary retention: rapid versus gradual decompression and risk of complications. *Mayo Clin Proc.* 1997;72(10):951.
7. Niel-Weise BS, Van Den Broek PJ. Antibiotic policies for short-term catheter bladder drainage in adults. *Cochrane Database Syst Rev.* 20 Juy 2005;(3):CD005428.
8. Caine M, Pfau A, Perlberg S. The use of alpha-adrenergic blockers in benign prostatic obstruction. *Br J Urol.* 1976;48(4):255.
9. Fisher E, Subramonian K, Omar MI. The role of alpha blockers prior to removal of urethral catheter for acute urinary retention in men. *Cochrane Database Syst Rev.* 10 June 2014;(6):CD006744.
10. McConnell JD, Bruskewitz R, Walsh P, et al. The effect of finasteride on the risk of acute urinary retention and the need for surgical treatment among men with benign prostatic hyperplasia. *N Engl J Med.* 1998;338(9):557.
11. Taube M, Gajraj H. Trial without catheter following acute retention of urine. *Br J Urol.* 1989;63(2):180.
12. Marshal JR, Haber J, Josephson EB. An evidence-based approach to emergency dept management of acute urinary retention. *Emerg Med Pract.* 2014;16:1.

79. NON-INVASIVE VENTILATION (BIPAP)

1. Rochwerg B, Brochard L, Elliott MW, et al. Official ERS/ATS clinical practice guidelines: noninvasive ventilation for acute respiratory failure. *Eur Respir J.* 31 August 2017;50(2):1602426.
2. Sweet DD, Naismith A, Keenan SP, et al. Missed opportunities for noninvasive positive pressure ventilation: a utilization review. *J Crit Care.* 2008;23(1):111.
3. American Thoracic Society, European Respiratory Society, European Society of Intensive Care Medicine, and Sociétéde Réanimation de Langue Française. International Consensus Conferences in Intensive Care Medicine: noninvasive positive pressure ventilation in acute respiratory failure. *Am J Respir Crit Care Med.* 1 January 2001;163(1):283-291.

80. VOMITING

1. Hasler WL, Chey WD. Nausea and vomiting. *Gastroenterology.* 2003;125(6):1860.
2. American Gastroenterological Association. American Gastroenterological Association medical position statement: nausea and vomiting. *Gastroenterology.* 2001;120(1):261.
3. Brzana RJ, Koch KL. Gastroesophageal reflux disease presenting with intractable nausea. *Ann Intern Med.* 1997;126(9):704.
4. Herrell HE. Nausea and vomiting of pregnancy. *Am Fam Physician.* June 2014;89(12):965-970.
5. Harrington BC, Jimerson M, Haxton C, et al. Initial evaluation, diagnosis, and treatment of anorexia nervosa and bulimia nervosa. *Am Fam Physician.* January 2015;91(1):46-52.
6. Quigley EM, Hasler WL, Parkman HP. AGA technical review on nausea and vomiting. *Gastroenterology.* January 2001;120(1):263-286.
7. Sack U, Biereder B, Elouahidi T, Bauer K, Keller T, Tröbs RB. Diagnostic value of blood inflammatory markers for detection of acute appendicitis in children. *BMC Surg.* 2006;6:15.
8. National Collaborating Centre for Women's and Children's Health (UK). *Diarrhea and Vomiting Caused by Gastroenteritis: Diagnosis, Assessment and Management in Children Younger than 5 Years. NICE Clinical Guidelines*, No. 84. London, UK: RCOG Press, 2009.
9. Koren G. Motherisk update. Is ondansetron safe for use during pregnancy? *Can Fam Physician.* October 2012;58(10):1092-1093.
10. [No authors listed]. Ondansetron looks safe in pregnancy, so far. *BMJ.* 6 March 2013;346:f1387.
11. Patanwala AE, Amini R, Hays DP, Rosen P. Antiemetic therapy for nausea and vomiting in the emergency department. *J Emerg Med.* September 2010;39(3):330-336.
12. Hines S, Steels E, Chang A, Gibbons K. Aromatherapy for treatment of postoperative nausea and vomiting. *Cochrane Database Syst Rev.* 18 April 2012;(4):CD007598.
13. Olden KW, Chepyala P. Functional nausea and vomiting. *Nat Clin Pract Gastroenterol Hepatol.* 2008;5(4):202.

81. WARFARIN OVERDOSE (SUPRATHERAPEUTIC INR)

1. Watt BE, Proudfoot AT, Bradberry SM, Vale JA. Anticoagulant rodenticides. *Toxicol Rev.* 2005;24(4):259.
2. Mullins ME, Brands CL, Daya MR. Unintentional pediatric superwarfarin exposures: do we really need a prothrombin time? *Pediatrics.* February 2000;105(2):402-404.
3. Bauman ME, Black K, Bauman ML, Kuhle S, Bajzar L, Massicotte MP. Warfarin induced coagulopathy in children: assessment of a conservative approach. *Arch Dis Child.* 2011;96(2):164.
4. Mahtani KR, Heneghan CJ, Nunan D, Roberts NW. Vitamin K for improved anticoagulation control in patients receiving warfarin. *Cochrane Database Syst Rev.* 15 May 2014;(5):CD009917.
5. Ansell J, Hirsh J, Hylek E, Jacobson A, Crowther M, Palareti G. Pharmacology and management of the vitamin K antagonists: American College of Chest Physicians Evidence-Based Clinical Practice Guidelines (8th Edition). *Chest.* 2008;133(6 Suppl):160S.
6. Fang MC, Go AS, Chang Y, et al. A new risk scheme to predict warfarin-associated hemorrhage: The ATRIA (Anticoagulation and Risk Factors in Atrial Fibrillation) Study. *J Am Coll Cardiol.* 2011;58(4):395.
7. Holbrook A, Schulman S, Witt DM, et al. Evidence-based management of anticoagulant therapy: antithrombotic therapy and prevention of thrombosis, 9th ed.: American College of Chest Physicians evidence-based clinical practice guidelines. *Chest.* February 2012;141(2 Suppl):e152S-e184S.
8. Garcia DA, Baglin TP, Weitz JI, Samama MM. Parenteral anticoagulants: antithrombotic therapy and prevention of thrombosis, 9th ed: American College of Chest Physicians evidence-based clinical practice guidelines. *Chest.* February 2012;141(2 Suppl):e24S-e43S.
9. Ansell J, Hirsh J, Hylek E, Jacobson A, Crowther M, Palareti G. Pharmacology and management of the vitamin K antagonists: American College of Chest Physicians evidence-based clinical practice guidelines (8th ed.). *Chest.* 2008;133(6 Suppl):160S.

3 Credit Line Listing

CHAPTER 3: ABG

Reprinted with permission from Chila AG. Foundations of Osteopathic Medicine. 3rd ed. Philadelphia: Wolters Kluwer Health; 2010. Fig. 59–2

CHAPTER 4: ACETAMINOPHEN OD

Reprinted with permission from Rumack BH, Matthew H. Acetaminophen poisoning and toxicity. *Pediatrics* 1975;55:871–876.

CHAPTER 5: ACLS CARDIAC ARREST

Figure 5.1. Reprinted with permission from Coviello JS. ECG Interpretation: *An Incredibly Easy Pocket Guide*. Philadelphia: Wolters Kluwer Health; 2017

Figure 5.2. Reprinted with permission from Coviello JS. ECG Interpretation: *An Incredibly Easy Pocket Guide*. Philadelphia: Wolters Kluwer Health; 2017.

Figure 5.3. Reprinted with permission from Coviello JS. ECG Interpretation: *An Incredibly Easy Pocket Guide*. Philadelphia: Wolters Kluwer Health; 2017.

CHAPTER 7: ACUTE CORONARY SYNDROME

Figure 7.1. Courtesy of Dr. Qiangjun Cai.

Table 7.1. Reproduced with permission from Six AJ, Backus BE, Kelder JC. *Chest pain in the emergency room: value of the HEART score*. Neth Heart J. 2008;16(6):191–196. Copyright © 2008 Bohn Stafleu van Loghum.

CHAPTER 22: C-SPINE INJURY

Data from: Hoffman JR et al. *Validity of a set of clinical criteria to rule out injury to the cervical spine in patients with blunt trauma*. National Emergency-Radiography Utilization Study Group. N Engl J Med 2000;343 and Stiell IG et al. The Canadian C-spine rule for radiography in alert and stable trauma patients. JAMA 2001;286:1841. In: Court-Brown CM, Heckman JD, McQueen MM, et al. *Rockwood and Green's Fractures in Adults*. Philadelphia: Wolters Kluwer Health; 2015.

CHAPTER 23: CVA

Courtesy of National Institute of Neurological Disorders and Stroke (NINDS)

CHAPTER 25: DENTAL ABSCESS

Reprinted with permission from Wilkins E. *Clinical Practice of the Dental Hygienist*. 12th ed. Philadelphia: Wolters Kluwer Health; 2017.

CHAPTER 79: VENT

Republished with permission of Daedalus Enterprises Inc. from Medoff BD. *Invasive and Noninvasive Ventilation in Patients With Asthma. Respir Care*. 2008;53(6):740–748; discussion 749–750; permission conveyed through Copyright Clearance Center, Inc.

Note: Page numbers followed by "*f*" and "*t*" refer to figures and tables, respectively.

Q

R